sleep meditations

**For Jamie and Georgia,
May your dreams be your
guiding force.
Oceans of love always xx**

An Hachette UK Company
www.hachette.co.uk

First published in Great Britain
in 2020 by Aster, an imprint of
Octopus Publishing Group Ltd
Carmelite House,
50 Victoria Embankment,
London EC4Y 0DZ
www.octopusbooks.co.uk

Text copyright © Danielle North 2020
Illustrations copyright © SpaceFrog
Designs 2020

Distributed in the US by
Hachette Book Group
1290 Avenue of the Americas,
4th and 5th Floors, New York,
NY 10104

Distributed in Canada by
Canadian Manda Group
664 Annette Street, Toronto,
Ontario, Canada M6S 2C8

ISBN 978 1 78325 357 9

A CIP catalogue record for this book
is available from the British Library.

Printed and bound in The Czech
Republic

10 9 8 7 6 5 4 3

Consultant Publisher: Kate Adams
Art Director: Yasia Williams-Leedham
Illustrators: SpaceFrog Designs
Senior Editor: Alex Stetter
Copy Editor: Caroline West
Production Manager: Lisa Pinnell

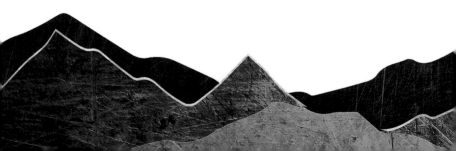

sleep meditations

to help tired minds unwind and drift off...

ASTER*

Danielle North

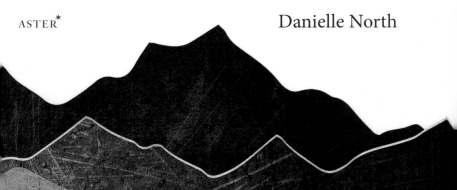

Contents

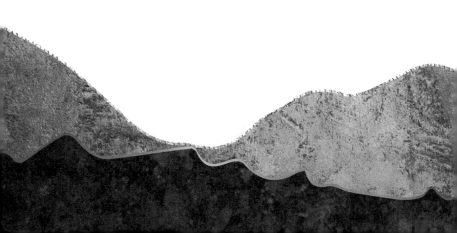

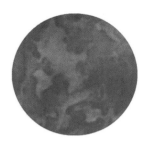

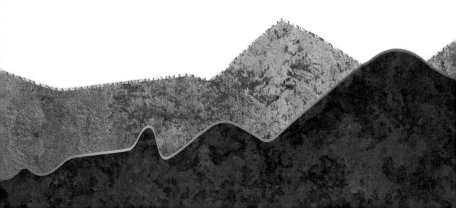

Introduction
Preparing for restful sleep

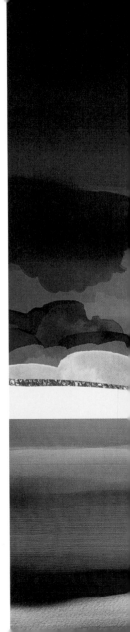

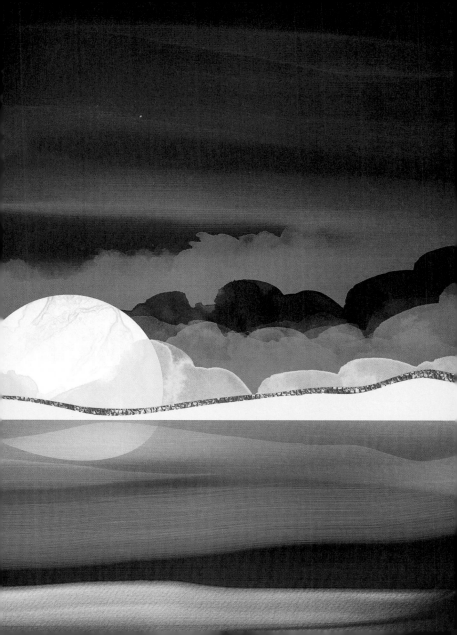

Sleep is such a precious thing, a time not only of rest, repair and rejuvenation, but also of a deep connection to ourselves through our dreams. Yet during the course of our lives we may find there are periods when our sleep is disturbed. An obvious time for this is during the transition to parenthood, but other factors such as exam stress, changes of season, ill health, work pressures and stimulants (for example caffeine, alcohol or sugar), or even just getting older, can all affect the quality of our sleep. Although it may seem obvious, how we sleep greatly affects our energy levels and our ability to focus, create and perform when we are awake.

Many people practise meditation as a morning ritual for clearing the mind in order to settle into the flow of the day. This is valuable and definitely recommended, but, as the busyness of the day takes over, we often give less

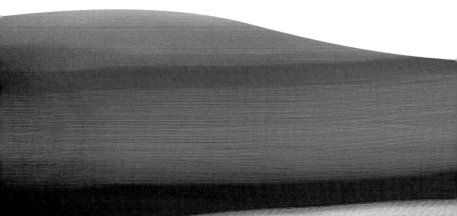

thought to the way we end our day and prepare for sleep. Most new mothers understand the significant benefits of a bedtime ritual for their baby; keeping a regular rhythm soothes babies and sends them to sleep – and the same is true for adults. Turning off electronic devices, turning down electric lights, reducing stimulants and generally preparing yourself for sleep will, over time, have a calming effect on your central nervous system, allowing you to get a peaceful and restorative night's sleep.

This book contains a series of meditations that are designed to relax you as you read them and bring you into the energy of rest. For each meditation there is a suggestion for an accompanying essential oil (or combination of oils), selected both to support the theme of the meditation and to aid sleep. Each meditation also begins with a short ritual before guiding you into a restful place.

Feel free to add these extra little touches if you wish, but the meditation is designed to work without them, so they are optional. Also explained is whether it is best to be standing, sitting or lying down for each meditation, but please make any necessary adjustments to suit your body. This book is also available in audio format if you would like to listen to the meditations.

Since these are sleep meditations, it is a good idea to be ready for bed when you have finished them. This way, you can retain the mental and emotional state gained from the meditation. Suggestions for preparing yourself include switching off your television, smartphone and any other electronic devices; shutting the curtains or blinds; and keeping the lights low by using candles so your melatonin levels are not disturbed.

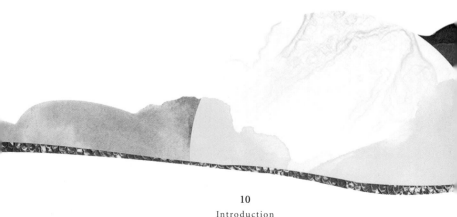

Aim to create a comfortable cocoon in your bedroom, whatever that might involve for you – some people like their bed to be made, while others prefer the sheets to be crumpled. Some people like a neat space, whereas others feel more relaxed having their things around them. Whatever your preference, make sure your bedroom feels inviting to you. Shut the curtains and put a low light on in this room as well, if it isn't the place you are going to be meditating.

Go someplace nice in your dreams.
Oceans of love,
Danielle x

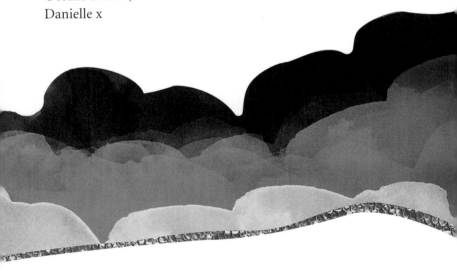

Essential oils

Essential oils not only smell wonderful but also have healing properties. Essential oils that might help you sleep include **lavender**, **bergamot** and **vetiver**. Try rubbing vetiver into the soles of your feet at bedtime and sprinkling lavender on your pillow; you can also mix a few drops into Epsom salts to add to your bath (see opposite). Put a few drops of both bergamot and lavender into a diffuser in your bedroom before you go to bed. I have included an accompanying essential oil for each meditation, but these are not needed for the meditation to work its magic – they are a little optional extra.

Here are three more of my favourite essential oils that I would recommend for tired minds:

✳ Basil: This oil is good for adrenal exhaustion and supports people who are feeling fatigued and overwhelmed. It is wonderful for giving optimism to tired souls.

* Cedarwood: A woody oil that will soothe an overworked mind and help you to feel grounded.

* Rose: This powerful oil is a heart-healer for emotional heartbreak. It is also a wonderful oil to use during meditation to help you connect to your love and compassion.

Note: Not all essential oils are suitable for pregnant women or children, so it is advisable to check this carefully before using. Where topical application (direct to skin) without a carrier oil is suggested, use only one to two drops. If you have sensitive skin, then always use a carrier oil. Almond oil or fractionated coconut oil work particularly well as carrier oils.

Epsom salts

Adding Epsom salts to a warm bath is a simple way to detox the body. The salts contain magnesium, which helps both the muscles and mind to relax. Epsom salts will raise your temperature slightly as part of their natural detoxifying process, so take that into account when adding them to your bath before bedtime.

Shake off the day

If you are feeling stiff, sluggish or stressed from your day, one of the simplest ways to re-energize is to shake. Start by giving yourself permission to switch off from your day for a few minutes. If you want to play some of your favourite music to put you in a good mood, then put it on now.

Slip off your shoes, loosen any tight belts or restrictive clothing and, when you are ready to begin, stand comfortably with your feet hip-width apart. Let your arms relax by your sides and become aware of your breathing. As you stand, feel your energy levels in this moment, right here, right now. How would you score your current energy levels on a scale of zero to ten? Are you flagging and finding it hard to support your body as you stand? If this is true for you, then choose a number at the lower end of the scale. If you have lots of energy and feel wide awake, then select a higher number, or perhaps you feel somewhere in the middle. Be honest with yourself, however you might be feeling in this moment.

Put the numbers to one side for now and begin by breathing a little more deeply into your belly. Place one hand on your chest and the other hand on your belly, and notice your breath as you inhale and exhale. Relax your arms and, as you breathe, begin to shake your body. Very gently at first. Let yourself shake from your fingertips, moving into your hands, shaking your wrists, still softy at this stage, just loosening off your wrists as you begin to feel the shaking travel up your arms and into your elbows. Increase the shaking so it moves up your arms and into your shoulders. Now both your arms are shaking – let them be free and fluid, and allow your body to shake in the way that suits you. If you want to shake more vigorously, and that feels OK, then begin to increase the intensity while remaining relaxed.

Let your shoulders, chest and torso shake now, bringing some movement into your head and neck so that the whole of your upper body is shaking. Let the shaking travel into your hips, circling, shaking and moving them, however they want to loosen up from the day.

Shake out your legs one at a time, lifting your foot off the ground to give your whole leg a good shake. With both feet back on the floor now, keep the upper body shaking while you let your thighs, knees, calves and ankles shake. Shake your body from the bottom to the top and back down again. Go as wild and crazy as you want, letting the energy build and rise.

Shake your face and, if you wish, make some sound – then you can shake yourself from the inside out! Have fun as you shake, smile, laugh, let go, be free. When you feel all shaken out, let your body begin to slow down, gradually coming back to your original standing position with your feet hip-width apart. Place one hand on your chest and the other on your belly again, and become aware of your breath as you inhale and exhale. Take a moment to check in. How are your energy levels now? They may be higher or lower. Let yourself trust whatever is true for you in this moment, right here, right now.

Grounding at the end of the day

During any given day your attention and focus can be split in a thousand different directions. Most of us attempt to multitask more than we realize. When your attention is divided like this, you might feel spaced out and distracted, or make mistakes. Over time, this builds up as you lose a sense of yourself and what you need. The further you move away from your centre, the more difficult it becomes to settle into periods of peaceful rest.

When you feel split like this, you may experience millions of thoughts rolling around like marbles in your mind. One way to bring yourself back to a balanced position, so you can rest well, is to practise grounding. The practice of grounding can take many forms. The intention is to harmonize your mind and emotions by connecting back to your body and, if possible, to the earth. Grounding is essentially like the earthing pin in a plug – a way of neutralizing the currents running through your system.

Some of the best ways to ground involve being in Nature, perhaps standing barefoot on grass, swimming in the ocean, sitting with your back nestled into the trunk of a tree or letting a river run through your heart. However, it is not always practical or possible to get grounded in Nature. So, when you need a way to get grounded in the comfort of your own home, try the yoga asana (pose) called Vrikshasana. Also known as Tree Pose, it doesn't require any previous yoga experience, but it does require concentration, balance and awareness, which is why it works so well for grounding.

Begin by removing your shoes and socks, and any tight belts or restrictive clothing. Stand with your feet close together, wiggle your toes and take a breath deep down into your belly, and then exhale. Repeat the breath six times, letting yourself sink more deeply into the ground with every exhale. Now adjust your feet, knees and hips so they are aligned. You will sway while you stand, that's natural – simply come back to an aligned position.

As you stand, begin to feel roots growing from the soles of your feet down into the earth beneath you.

As you breathe, let your body be both firm and relaxed, with your roots going down into the ground and the crown of your head stretching your whole spine skywards.

When you are ready, pour all of your rooted energy into your left leg, and lightly lift your right foot. Place the sole of your right foot on the inside of your left leg wherever feels comfortable (avoiding the knee). Focus your gaze on a point in front of you and continue to breathe and pour your rooted energy into your left leg. If you are able, bring your hands into a prayer position at your heart centre. If you sway or wobble, that's OK – just come back to your starting position and begin again.

When you are ready, return to your original position and then repeat the asana, this time pouring your energy into your right leg and lightly lifting your left leg.

When you are in the asana, remember to focus your attention on the crown of your head, so you can lift your spine and head skywards while also feeling your roots going into the ground.

Breathe easy

This is a simple breathing exercise for calming both the nervous system and an overworked mind. It's a breath where the exhale is longer than the inhale. When your exhale is even a few counts longer than your inhale, the vagus nerve, which runs from the neck to the diaphragm, sends a signal to your brain to turn up your parasympathetic nervous system and turn down your sympathetic nervous system.

For many of us, modern living activates the sympathetic nervous system and our cortisol levels become elevated for too long, creating a hormonal imbalance that makes it difficult to switch off. When the parasympathetic nervous system is activated, your breathing slows, your heart rate drops, your blood pressure lowers and your body is put into a state of calm. You can use this breathing practice to let go of the stresses, strains and challenges of the day, to leave you feeling relaxed and light.

Begin sitting in a comfortable position and, as you get settled, check in with how you are feeling. Will you be OK with where you are right now?

Notice the weight of your body in the seat. Let yourself relax as much as you can. If you are sitting on a chair, put your feet on the floor and rest your hands gently in your lap. Know that this is your time. Hold your spine straight and allow your head to rest easy, allowing the muscles around your eyes to relax. Then tuck your chin ever so slightly towards your neck. Let your jaw relax; your mouth might be slightly open and the tip of your tongue gently touching the front roof of your mouth.

If you notice your mind is busy, that's OK. Just allow the thoughts to come and go; they won't interfere with what you are doing here. Begin to notice your breath, the inhale and exhale. Become aware of the air naturally entering your body and naturally leaving. Notice how your breath is today. Is it shallow, is it deep, where does it naturally want to go? Can you be with your breath just as it is for now? There is no need to change it or alter it in this moment.

Now gently begin to deepen your inhale, breathing in through your nose, down into your belly and out through your mouth, as if you are blowing out a candle. This is called a conscious breath. Repeat that one more time: breathe in through your nose, down into your belly and out through your mouth as if you're blowing out a candle.

On the next breath, your exhale is going to be two counts longer than your inhale. As you inhale, you might count to four and then, as you exhale, you might count to six. Try that now to see how a count of four suits you: as you inhale, count to four and as you exhale count to six. Each person's breath is different, so experiment with the count that suits you, and find your own rhythm. You can't get this wrong because everybody is unique – it's just counting and breathing.

Let yourself settle into your own breathing rhythm, where your exhale is two counts longer than your inhale.

If you can, at the top of your inhale, pause for a second before you exhale. So, you inhale for a count of four, pause, and then exhale for a count of six. Inhale for four, pause, exhale for six. Keep going with the breathing, and settle into your count, your rhythm and your breath.

As you breathe, become aware of your body and let any tension go on the out breath, with your exhale being two counts longer than your inhale. As you exhale, let go of any tension in your eyes. Exhale, letting go of any tension in your jaw. On the next exhale, let go of any tension in your shoulders, then let go on of any tension in your stomach. Now let go of any tension in your legs. On the next exhale, soften your whole body.

Now you're going to return to a normal breath. No counts, no longer exhales, no pauses – just letting your breath do what it naturally does. As you return to your natural breath, notice how you feel now. What is happening with your body? Can you be with it all, just as it is?

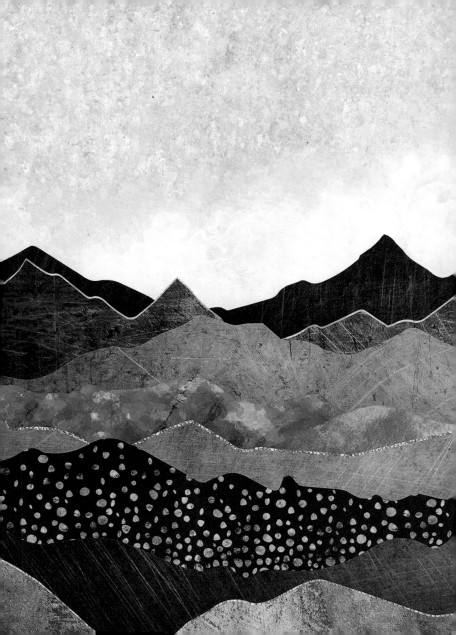

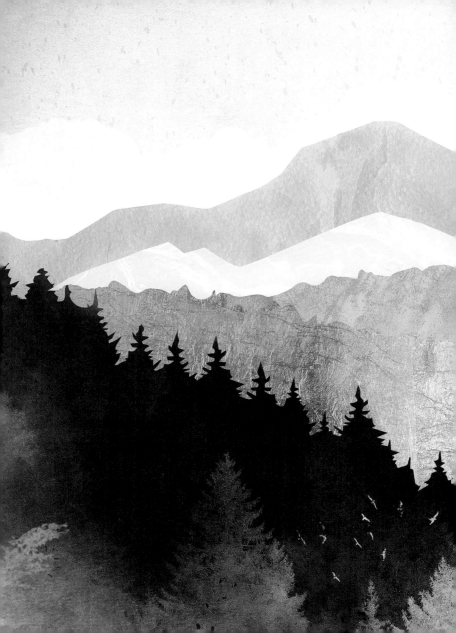

* Evening meditations

The bridge to…

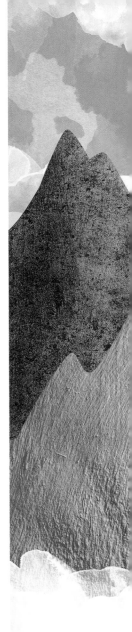

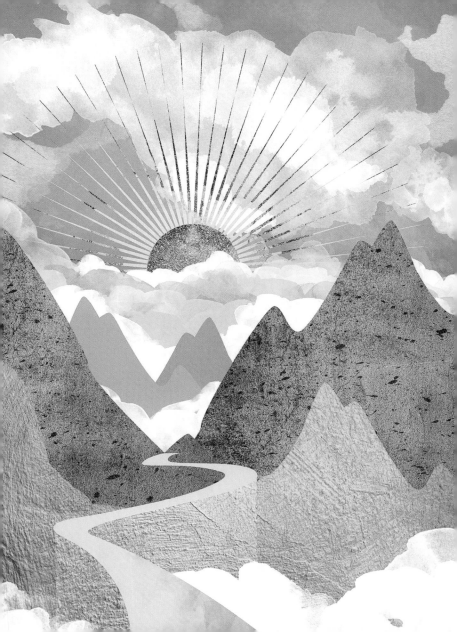

* Essential oil: Mix one to two drops of clary sage essential oil with a carrier oil and apply it to your forehead before beginning the meditation to help you imagine new possibilities.

* Ritual: Turn off your smartphone, find your notebook or journal, and spend a few minutes writing about what is good in your life right now. Next, spend a few more minutes writing about a change you would like to make. This could be a physical or environmental change; it might be an emotional change or perhaps it is a shift in your perception – whatever you feel would enhance your quality of life at this time. For the purpose of this exercise, focus on just one change so you don't overstimulate your mind.

✳ Set up your meditation space as you would like it; this is
a standing meditation and you will need to make sure there
is enough space in front of you to take about five steps with
no obstacles in your way.

If you are wearing shoes, remove them now. Stand with your
feet hip-width apart, wiggle your toes and make contact with
the floor beneath you.

Take a moment to move your body and loosen off any areas of tension.

Wriggle your hips, scrunch your shoulders, shake your arms
and legs, and open your mouth to release your jaw. Now take
a deep inhale in through your nose and let it travel right down
into your belly. As you exhale, let out a sigh or any sound that
feels good to you right now. Repeat three times. This deep
breathing can assist with the relaxation process.

Return to your starting position and wait a moment for your breath to return to a regular rhythm. Lower your gaze and relax your body and mind for a couple of minutes.

Think about a change you would like to make in your life. Something that would enhance your quality of life or your wellbeing if you achieved it.

Make the change a bit of a stretch, but not something that is entirely out of reach – something that would be possible for you to attain. Take a moment to think about where you are now in relation to that change.

Now focus your gaze about five steps in front of you and picture the change you want to achieve. Imagine how life would be with this change in place in your life.

From the place where you are standing, visualize a beautiful bridge that leads you to your future vision. You are going to step onto this bridge and, with each step, you are going to consider what might need to happen for you to get a little closer to your vision. If space allows, you can physically take the steps (keeping your eyes open!) across the bridge.

With each step, take your time and consider what needs to happen for you to get a little closer.

Count the steps as you go: step one, step two, step three, step four, step five, until you reach the place of your future vision.

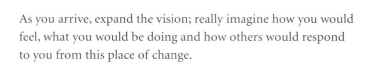

As you arrive, expand the vision; really imagine how you would feel, what you would be doing and how others would respond to you from this place of change.

Now look back at the bridge and consider what you need to let go of and what you need to let in along the way.

Thank your future self for having the courage to imagine new possibilities.

Then walk back across the bridge in the knowledge that where you are now is OK.

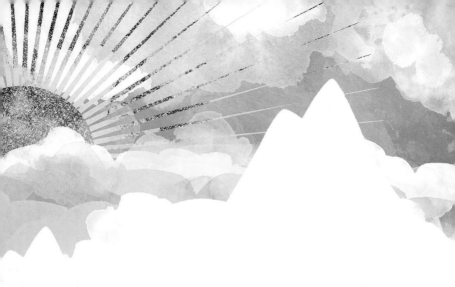

As you stand in your current reality, look over the bridge towards
your vision and let yourself know three qualities or gifts you
have that will enable you to cross this bridge over time.

Now stand with your feet hip-width apart and wiggle your toes
as you make contact with the floor beneath you.

Put your right hand on your left shoulder, and your left hand
on your right shoulder, and give yourself a really big hug.

Healing heart

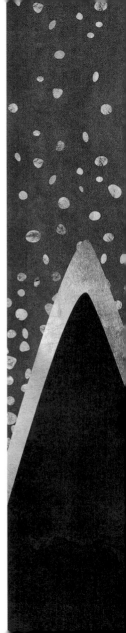

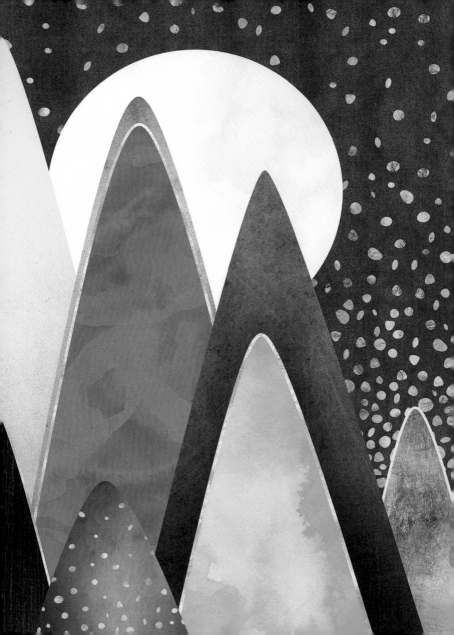

✳ **Essential oil:** To assist with emotional healing, add a mix of rose and geranium essential oils to a diffuser.

✳ **Ritual:** This ritual uses scented salts, and is lovely before and during your meditation, allowing you to sink more deeply into your healing. You can prepare the salts in advance as they will store well.

Find a large bowl into which you can comfortably fit both feet. Add one cup of Epsom salts or coarse sea salt to a mixing bowl, then stir in ten drops of rose essential oil and eight drops of geranium essential oil until everything is well mixed.

Put a towel on the floor where you would like to sit, then place the bowl on top. Fill the bowl with warm (not boiling) water, then add a quarter of a cup of your scented salts to the water. You can save the rest in a clean screw-top jar to use in a bath or foot soak another day. Soak your feet for ten to fifteen minutes before or during your meditation.

✳ Sit in a way that allows you to feel comfortable and relaxed. Make your breathing normal as you turn your attention inwards. Notice how you are feeling. Is there any physical tension or discomfort in your body? What is your emotional state? Are there any adjustments you would like to make to feel more comfortable right now?

If you have been busy during the day – and busy doesn't need to mean physically busy, as we can also be mentally or emotionally busy – then when you come to sit and meditate, all the feelings you weren't aware of can rise to the surface. Meditation doesn't cause these feelings. However, when you slow down and shift your focus from the outside world to your inner world, you become more aware of what was already present within you. There may be pain, sadness or loss. You may be aware of resentment, jealousy or anger. Sometimes these feelings are tiny, almost unnoticeable, but other times they can feel like a torrent threatening to engulf you. Whether your experience is subtle or overwhelming, these feelings are all signs that your heart has been hurt.

So, with all that in mind, however you are is OK. There is no need to alter anything unless it makes you feel more comfortable, in which case go ahead.

To enable you to relax even more deeply, you are going to count your breaths. An inhale and an exhale will count as one cycle of breath, and you are going to complete ten cycles. You can count each cycle of breath on your fingers. When you inhale, let the breath go in through your nose. When you exhale, let the breath leave your body through your mouth. It helps to have your lips parted so the breath can flow out easily.

Gently turn your attention to your breath.

When you are ready, begin to count ten cycles of breath. Remember, one cycle is an inhale through your nose and an exhale through your open mouth. Relax as you breathe in, and relax as you breathe out.

With every breath, let yourself relax even more deeply. If you lose count, don't worry, just start again. If you overshoot ten cycles, just stop when you realize. Try to stay present, awake and relaxed as you count.

Once you have completed ten cycles of breath, let the counting go and allow your breath to return to its regular rhythm.

If you feel yourself tensing up at any time, you can simply take one or two more cycles of breath.

You are going to let your attention rest on your heart by placing your right hand over your heart and turning your eyes inwards, in the direction of your heart. As you breathe, let the inhale and exhale come from beneath your hand.

When you are ready, let yourself connect to any feelings or sensations in your heart. Your experience might be mixed, but that's OK. Remember, sorrow and joy are often woven together.

Let yourself stay open to the experience of your own heart.

Some emotions might want to be expressed; if that is how you are feeling, then let them flow in whatever way suits you.

If it feels right, you might want to ask your heart a question; if one arises, trust your instincts.

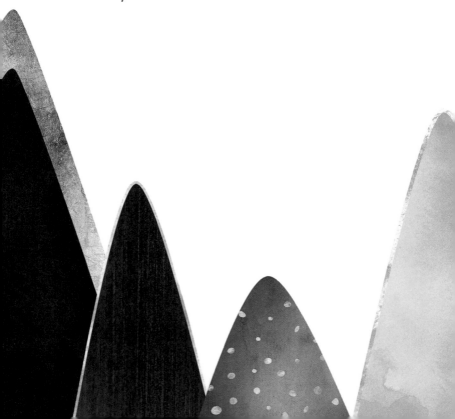

When you are ready, you can say this shortened version of the Buddhist Loving-Kindness meditation:

May I be happy.

May I be well.

May I be safe.

May I be peaceful and at ease.

You can say this as many times as you wish, letting the words permeate your heart.

You are now going to finish the meditation by closing your eyes and counting ten cycles of breath. As before, you can count each cycle on your fingers. The inhale is through your nose and the exhale is through your open mouth. An inhale and an exhale is one cycle. You can count the cycles in your own time.

When you have finished, let go of the counting and gently open your eyes as your breath returns to its regular rhythm.

Candle gazing

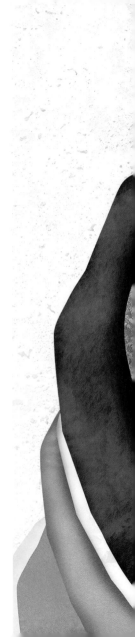

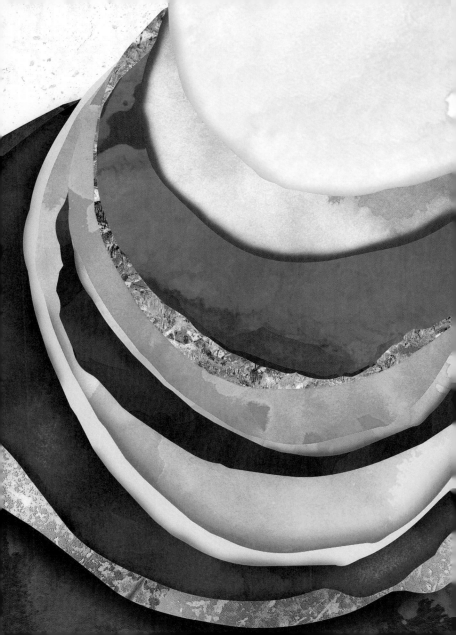

✳ Essential oil: To connect to your inner light during this meditation, add some melissa essential oil to a diffuser or mix one to two drops with a carrier oil, rub into the palms of your hands and inhale.

✳ Ritual: Set your space by lighting some candles. If you have them, bring your favourite crystals into the meditation space, arranging them around the candles. If you are new to crystals and would like to use one, you could begin with clear quartz, which you can hold lightly in your hands during the meditation. Close the curtains or blinds, switch off your smartphone and dim the lights. If you would like some gentle music in the background for this meditation, play that now.

✳ This is a seated meditation. If you have a candle, place it in a safe position in front of you.

During the meditation you can soften your gaze and watch the flame flicker.

Try not to blink too often and keep your gaze as soft as possible. If you don't have a candle, then, when the time comes, you can bring the image of a flame or a fire into your mind's eye.

To begin, sit in a position that is comfortable for you. Support your back if you wish, so your spine can be straight and you feel as comfortable as possible.

Become aware of your head supported on your shoulders and gently move your head from left to right six times. Return your head to the centre and now nod your head in a 'yes' movement forwards and backwards six times.

Now, keeping your shoulders relaxed, tip your left ear to your left shoulder, feel the stretch and then come back to the centre, before tipping your right ear to your right shoulder. Slowly repeat six times.

Next, circle your head in front of you, from left to right, and then from right to left six times.

Finally, shrug your shoulders up to your ears six times and then return your head to the centre.

Wriggle your jaw to release any tension here, and then tip your chin slightly towards your chest.

Blink your eyes firmly six times, then begin to soften the muscles around your forehead, letting the muscles around your eyes relax and soften.

Imagine a space between your eyes and breathe deeply into this space.

Now, either look at your candle flame with soft eyes or imagine a flame or fire in your mind's eye.

Keep your soft focus on the flame and begin to observe what you see. Notice the movement, the colours, and the light and shade within the flame. Let the flame guide you. What else do you see?

Now imagine there is a flame within you, an inner light.

Let your attention rest on your own inner light, your inner beauty. What do you notice here? Let the goodness of your own inner light grow and expand. See how brightly you can shine. Become aware of the quality of your light.

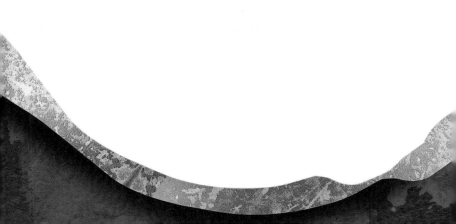

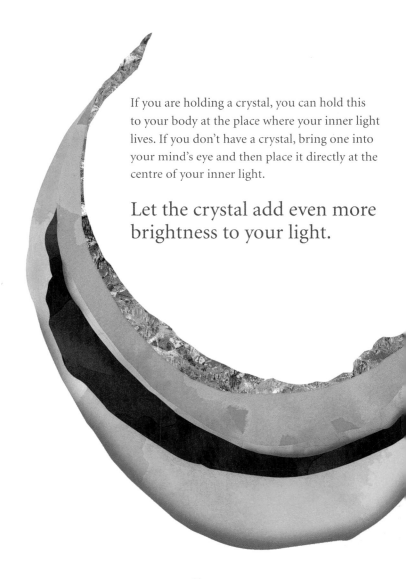

If you are holding a crystal, you can hold this to your body at the place where your inner light lives. If you don't have a crystal, bring one into your mind's eye and then place it directly at the centre of your inner light.

Let the crystal add even more brightness to your light.

Allow a kaleidoscope of colour to dance from the crystal and watch the many dimensions that open up within your light. Let the flame dance within the crystal, as the flame and the crystal become one source of light within you.

Now imagine the light surrounds your entire being, infusing every cell, enveloping you and protecting you.

When you are ready, return your focus to the original flame.

Watch the flame dance and flicker, seeing the colours and beauty within it, as you return to the natural rhythm of your breath.

Maybe it's magic

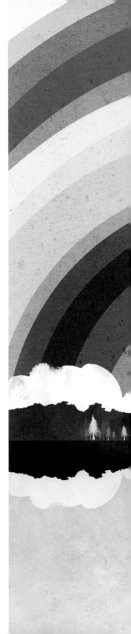

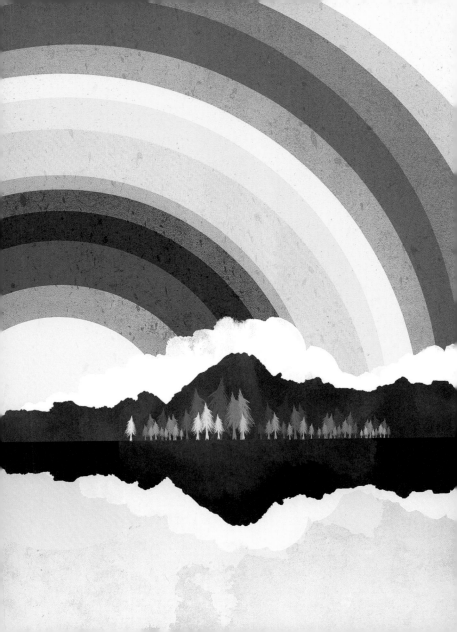

✳ Essential oil: To help you stay rooted during this meditation, mix three to four drops of cedarwood essential oil with a carrier oil and apply it to the soles of your feet.

✳ Ritual: Clear the energy of your space with a technique known as smudging. To do this, light a stick of palo santo and then walk around, allowing the fragrant smoke to waft into the top and bottom corners of the room, relighting the palo santo stick as needed. Alternatively, you can use a singing bowl or chimes, if you have them, and clear the energy of the space using sound. Choose a corner at the top of the room, then work your way around the space in a spiral and end at a corner in the bottom of the room. You can move in any direction and keep going until you feel ready to stop. Light some incense and turn down the lights.

✳ If you have a meditation cushion, sit on that; otherwise any
cushion will do. For most people, being raised up slightly
allows them to sit in a cross-legged position more comfortably
and for longer. If you need to support your back during the
meditation, put the cushion next to a wall so you can keep
your spine straight.

Prepare by sitting cross-legged on your cushion, with your
spine straight but not rigid. Tip your chin slightly towards
your chest to open the channel at the base of your neck.

Lower your gaze and rest your hands on your knees.

If you wish, you can connect the thumb and forefinger of both hands to complete the energy circuit.

Become aware of the movement of breath in your upper chest.
On the next inhale, let your breath fill your side ribs, expanding
them outwards. As you inhale, become aware of your breath in
your solar plexus. Now, on your next inhale, let the breath fill
your abdomen.

Reverse this now: first focus on filling your abdomen.
Then inhale into your solar plexus. Now inhale and expand
your side ribs.

On the next inhale, become aware of the breath in your upper
chest. Let your breath settle into its natural rhythm and, in your
mind's eye, visualize a rainbow forming, one colour at a time.

First you see the **violet** arc, then an **indigo** arc. A **blue** arc comes next, followed by a **green**, then a **yellow**, an **orange** and, finally, a **red** arc completes the entire rainbow.

You gaze in wonder at the pure beauty of this magical creation.

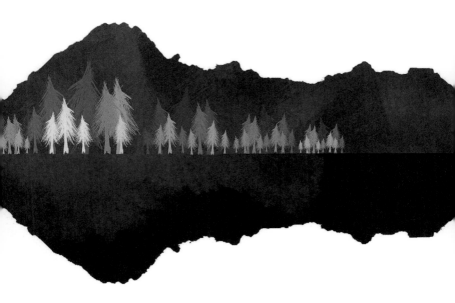

Maybe it's magic

Now you are going to infuse each of these colours into the seven chakras, or energy centres, of your own being, one by one.

Starting with a deep and powerful **red** light, feel the energy of the light run down your spine and gather at the base, your root chakra. Here, as you pour bright red energy into the base of your spine, you connect to your fundamental need for stability. As you flood your root chakra with deep red light, you begin to feel more grounded and rooted.

Then, vivid **orange** energy fills your abdomen, lighting up your sacral chakra just below your navel. As you let the vivid orange energy flow, you watch a multitude of different tones and hues of orange dance and change, swirling in a beautiful mix within your sacral chakra, with every breath expanding your connection to your creativity.

Now breathe into your solar plexus chakra, the area above your navel, and fill this space with bright **yellow** energy. Visualize the happiest, brightest yellow energy filling you with pure and radiant clarity, which sources and powers you.

Move your attention to your heart chakra and visualize a river of **green** energy flowing into your heart. The river runs softly into your heart, and the green light fills your heart, holds your heart and opens your heart. As your heart is infused with the green light, you feel more emotionally connected, as new love for yourself and others is encouraged to grow.

As you move from your heart, you rest at your throat chakra, which fills with a brilliant, clear **blue** energy from the sea and the sky. You let the brilliant blue energy enter your throat chakra, encouraging clear and kind communication, the expression of your truest self.

Now you move to your third eye chakra, the space between your eyes.

You rest here for a while and let a delicate, soft **indigo** energy infuse your third eye chakra. As the light gradually enters your third eye, you watch the delicate indigo light become richer and deeper, enhancing your ability to connect with your own insight and intuition.

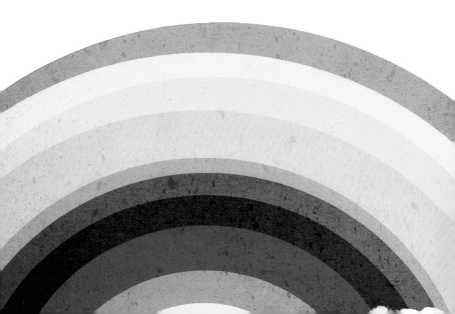

The final arc from your rainbow is a transformational **violet** energy, which pours in through the top of your head. As the violet light flows through your crown chakra, you watch it turn from its core into pure white light. This violet-white flame of light penetrates your entire being and connects you to the heavens.

You feel the wonder and possibility of your creation as you bathe in pure white light, connected through your whole being to the oneness that is ever present.

When you are ready, place your hands together at your heart centre and give thanks in a way that feels best for you.

Leaves settle

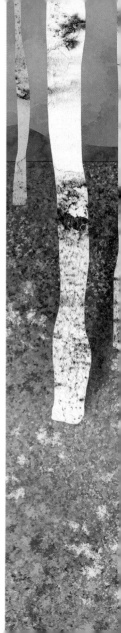

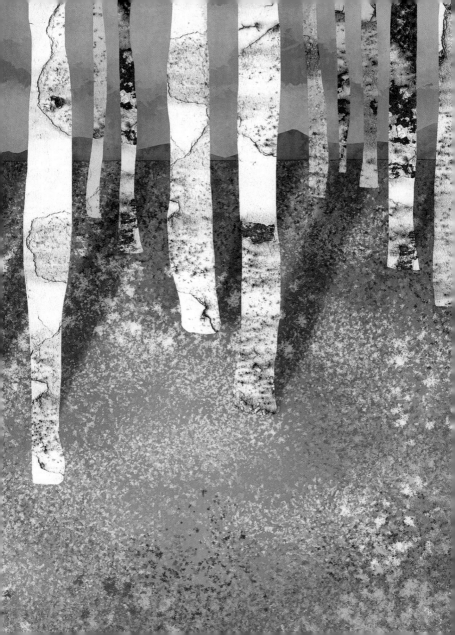

✲ Essential oil: To support this meditation, add some frankincense essential oil (known as the oil of truth) to a diffuser, or light some frankincense incense instead.

✲ Ritual: Perform a smudging ritual by lighting a white sage stick to cleanse the space and your own aura (energy field) for a few minutes. When you are ready, put the sage stick out, turn down the lights and sit in a comfortable position.

✳ You are going to take some time, just for you to cleanse your mind, to ease any overthinking so you can relax and rest. Begin by focusing on your breath. Notice the inhale and the exhale. Don't try to change them or alter them; for the next few breaths, just notice them.

Now, on your next inhale, picture a swirl of leaves playing in the wind.

The leaves are different shapes and sizes. You can see different colours, textures and patterns in the leaves. As you inhale, the leaves gently swirl and, as you exhale, the leaves slow down and settle. Repeat this ten times, letting the leaves gently swirl as you inhale and slow down and settle as you exhale. Each time the leaves settle you feel yourself slowing down, and your whole body and mind settles too. Take your time, settling deeper into yourself with every exhale.

Let yourself sink deeper and deeper, becoming more and more relaxed.

On your next inhale, follow your breath up through your nostrils and into your head. Let your attention linger here for a moment – in your beautiful mind that knows so much, yet remains curious and open to learn more.

The mind can be a busy place, and you may have thoughts in your mind that are unkind, or critical or judgemental. Even if they are not present now, it is likely you have heard them before. For now, notice or remember them, then observe them without pushing them away or attaching to them.

The thoughts may be about you, or others, or both. Simply notice the thoughts. On the next inhale imagine these thoughts swirling with the leaves in the wind. You can let them swirl at any speed you feel comfortable with, perhaps slowing the swirling down, or maybe speeding it up. Keep your breathing

steady until the thoughts become the leaves swirling and dancing gently in the wind. When you are ready, inhale and then exhale so that the leaves and the thoughts settle.

As the leaves and thoughts settle, for the next five breaths take a deep inhale and say, 'I am loved.' When you let the exhale out, say, 'You are loved.'

Now let it all go.

Let your breathing return to its normal rhythm. Notice the inhale and the exhale. Don't try to change them or alter them; for the next few breaths, just notice them. When you are ready, gently open your eyes.

If you wish, close with the smudging ritual and a herbal tea.

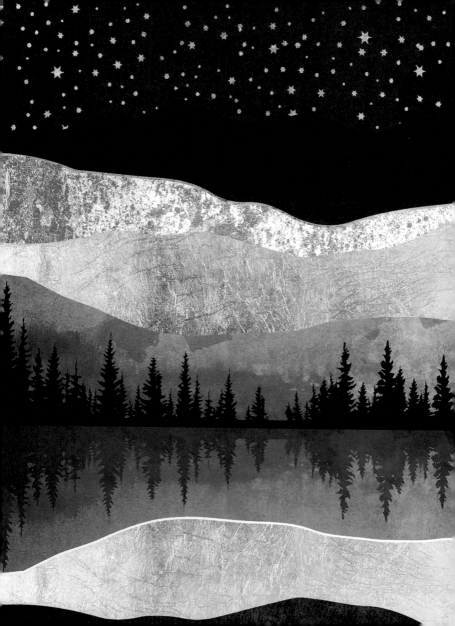

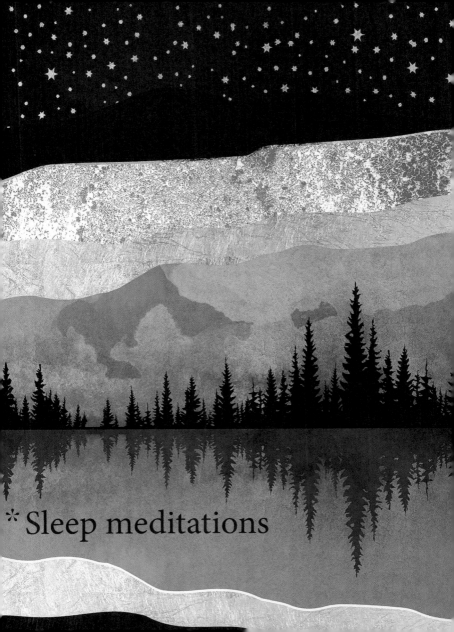

* Sleep meditations

Soul gathering

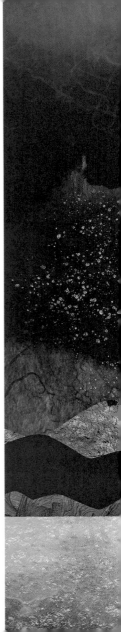

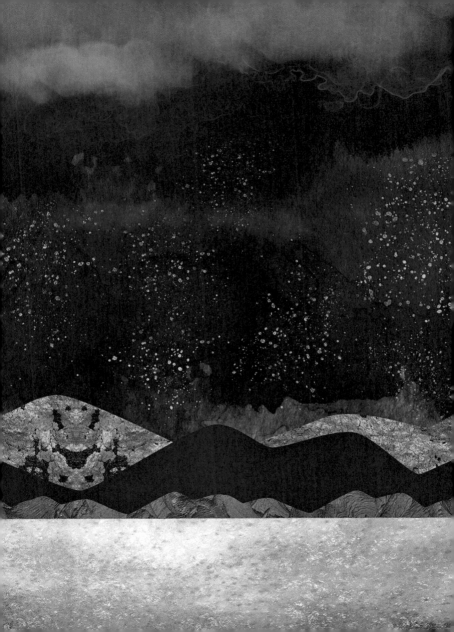

✳ Essential oil: To support this meditation, mix two drops of myrrh essential oil with a carrier oil and apply it over your heart. This will help you let go of fear.

✳ Ritual: Turn the lights down and lie on your back with your arms by your sides and your feet uncrossed. You can cover yourself with a blanket if you want extra warmth. As you settle down and your breathing begins to soften, take a moment to connect with your heart and the goodness within you. Choose one quality that you love about yourself, then amplify the energy of this quality and feel it radiate throughout your entire being.

✳ You have been on a journey, from the time you were born and even before then. Along the way, you have gained so much: love, insight, knowledge, friendship, perspective, confidence, understanding, wisdom and more. You have made memories that will stay with you for all eternity. However, the journey of your life has not always been an easy one, and there have been times along the way when you have lost parts of you, or perhaps you put the most precious parts of you in a safe place when they needed protection.

This is a meditation to gather back the lost parts of you, to bring your soul safely back home so that you can feel peaceful and whole.

During this meditation, it is important to let yourself feel any emotions that surface; now is the time and space for you to feel deeply and fully.

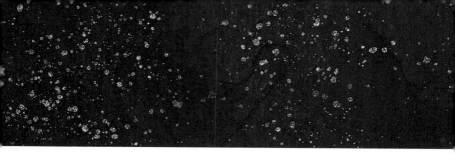

Become aware of the edges of your body connecting to the surface beneath you. Breathe deeply, inhaling and exhaling three times.

On each exhale, let yourself sink more deeply into the surface beneath you.

As you sink more deeply, you begin to let go, feeling the muscles in your face soften. As your jaw begins to soften, the tiny muscles around your eyes soften, then the space between your eyes softens. You are letting your throat soften now, as your tongue softens.

Feel your mind softening as your neck softens and your shoulders begin to soften and melt away beneath you. Your spine softens, and your chest expands and softens with every gentle breath you take. Your arms soften, your hands that work so hard soften completely, and every finger softens. Feel your heart soften, softening your breath down into your soft belly.

As you let your buttocks soften, your thighs soften. Even your knees soften now as your calves soften, your ankles soften and finally your toes soften.

Now your whole body softens; everything inside you softens and the edges of you soften as you breathe softly, completely letting go.

As you lie here, feeling soft, you remember the journey you have taken to reach this place in time. Your attention drifts to the people you have met, the loves and losses, the memories that matter the most to you. You let yourself be guided to people and places as they arise, not lingering too long to make sense of why they appear, simply trusting that everything is and always has unfolded as it is meant to.

Your attention drifts to you now, and the qualities within you, and what it has taken for you to make this journey in life, to be at this place in time. You are able to acknowledge your patience, your generosity, your courage, your love, your playfulness, your wisdom, your devotion, your dignity, your fierceness, your light, and your big, big heart. You know that you have not been these things at all times, in all situations, to all people, but that is OK. These qualities live within you.

You deserve to be acknowledged for the imperfectly perfect being you are.

Your attention drifts to the parts of you that you have needed to protect. You recall the moments that you closed off, shut down or split off parts of you. There is no judgement here; you did what was needed to protect and take good care of yourself.

Now is the time to remember what you have put where, and to consider if now would be a good time to dissolve the defences or call back those lost parts of you. Take your time, let your attention drift; you know where to look, just trust yourself.

You begin to absorb the lost parts of you, dissolving defences and returning parts that are ready to return. You notice there is a part of you that is far, far away. Perhaps it is being stored safely beyond this world in a different time and place. From the centre of your being you send out a fine silvery thread to this lost part of you. The thread is eternal and can cross time, space and dimensions. It knows just where to go to connect with the lost part of you. As the thread connects to the part of you that you are ready to retrieve, you feel a gentle tug at the centre of your being. You know it is time, and carefully, gently, you bring the silver thread back into the centre of your being.

As you gently bring the silver thread all the way into your core, you feel a light breeze dancing across your skin and you know all is well – you feel whole, safe and secure. From this place, your attention drifts to a question and you ask yourself:

What will it take to live from the centre of my being?

You consider the conditions your soul requires and, when you have contemplated this question, you thank yourself for all that you have been and all that you are. You infuse your whole being with love and gratitude.

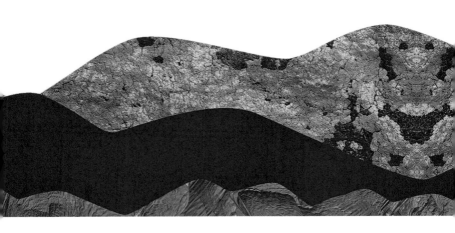

Your attention drifts back to your breath, the inhale and exhale. As you become aware of your breathing, you begin to notice your body, feeling the edges of you again and becoming aware of the edges of you connecting with the surface beneath you.

Take some time to feel the whole of you connecting to the surface beneath you.

Begin to wiggle your fingers and toes, letting some life gently enter you. When you are ready, roll onto your right side. From here, you can either press yourself up into a seated position or simply drift off to sleep.

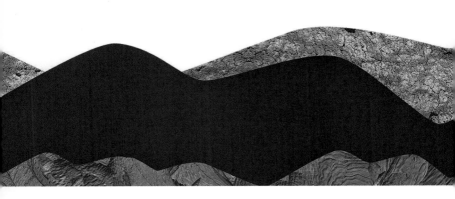

The easy path

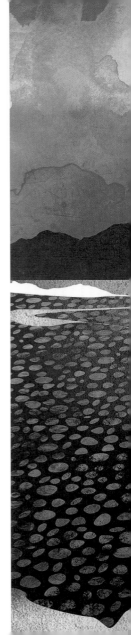

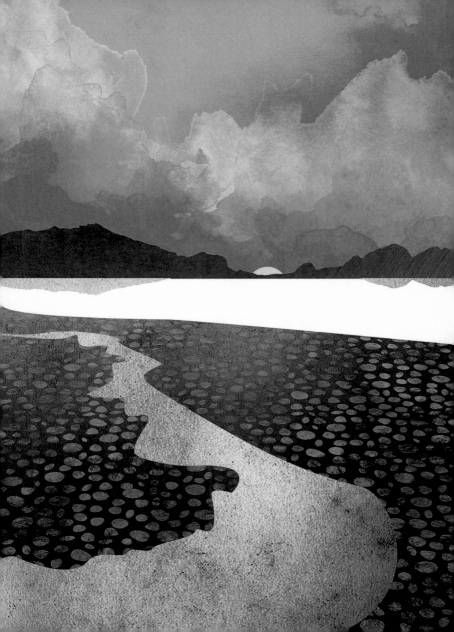

✳ Essential oil: To assist your meditation, mix one drop of sandalwood essential oil with a carrier oil and apply it to the crown of your head, or light some sandalwood incense.

✳ Ritual: Begin by going outside for a mindful walk for about ten to fifteen minutes. Leave your smartphone behind and be conscious of your surroundings. If possible, stand barefoot in the grass to get grounded. When you return home, turn the lights down low before you begin your meditation.

✳ Tonight you are going for a walk, which you know will follow the easy path. As you walk, you may see signs along the way. If you do, pay attention and trust your instincts.

Begin by relaxing your body for a minute or two. There is nothing to do except be here.

Become aware of your feelings and allow them to come to a restful place. Then consciously let your thoughts slow down with each breath until your mind feels relatively still.

You are standing at the base of a mountain. Although you are on your own, you know that you will be guided along the way, as you understand deep within that you are never really alone. You look up in awe at the majestic mountain as her summit breaks through the clouds. You know this mountain has witnessed much, endured great changes and continues to stand strong and steadfast.

The air is cool and you feel the mountain mist lightly touching your skin. You are aware that the sun's rays will slowly sink behind the skyline as you progress. You take a moment to fully appreciate your surroundings, hearing the sounds of nature all around you and deeply inhaling the pure mountain air. You can smell the rich aroma of the leaves beneath your feet. The earth is alive and awake to the warmth of the evening sun.

And then you step onto the path that is before you.

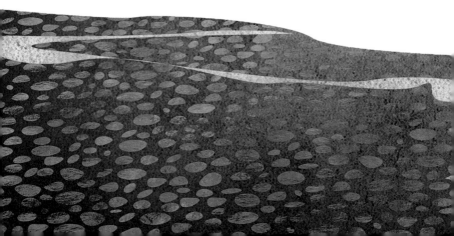

Although you are climbing a mountain, the path never feels strenuous and, as you continue your ascent, you realize that there is no need to push, to strive or to conquer this mountain – and that this has always been the case. You can sense the mountain supporting you as your feet make contact with the earth beneath them, encouraging you every step of the way. As you continue to follow the path, you remember that you have been here before, following the easy path as it reveals itself to you step by step. You realize that you can take your time and enjoy the journey; there really is no need to hurry at all.

All is well.

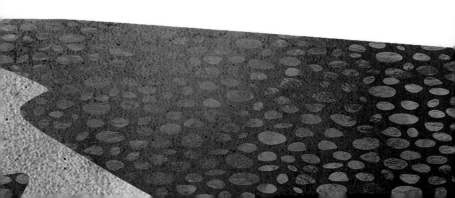

As you approach the summit and the ascent steepens, you slow down and allow your breathing to deepen. Fill your lungs with pure mountain air, remembering that the essentials of life are simply to inhale and exhale.

You sense that someone is waiting for you beyond the clouds. You do not know who, but in your heart you already know that you will be pleased to see them.

You take some time to pause and take in the view – it is the most magnificent vista, overlooking smaller mountains. You can see rivers meandering like molten threads of silver towards a lake that glistens in the sunlight.

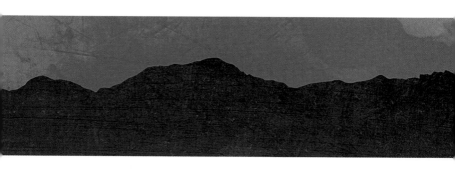

Your heart feels full, and you continue the final few steps through the clouds to the summit.

It is as though you have travelled into another world. A magical place, where time no longer exists and where love is ever-present.

Sitting on a rock with their back to you is a figure. Even though you cannot see their face, you know immediately who it is. You approach them and, as they turn to greet you, no words are spoken. Your eyes are able to transmit and receive all the love you both feel for one another. You take each other's hands and gaze into each other's eyes for what feels like an eternity.

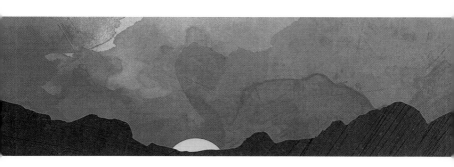

The easy path

It is almost time to leave, but before you do, your guide reaches into a bag and offers you a gift, an object that will help you to remember that the easy path is always available to you. You receive the gift wholeheartedly and say your wordless goodbyes.

Your guide sits back on the rock and you turn peacefully towards the path that is in front of you.

You understand now that it is your path and that no one else can walk it for you.

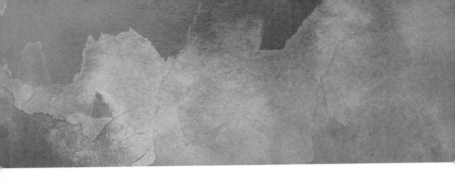

Make your way through the clouds and begin your descent with lightness in your steps.

Step by step, you follow the easy path back to the base of the mountain. You feel the mountain support you as she has always done, as the sun lowers and deepens into a rosy pink.

You know that although this is your path you will be guided along the way.

As you reach the foot of the mountain, you take a moment to look back up to where you have been and give thanks.

Still lake

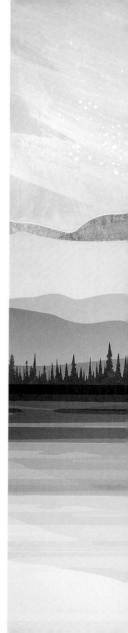

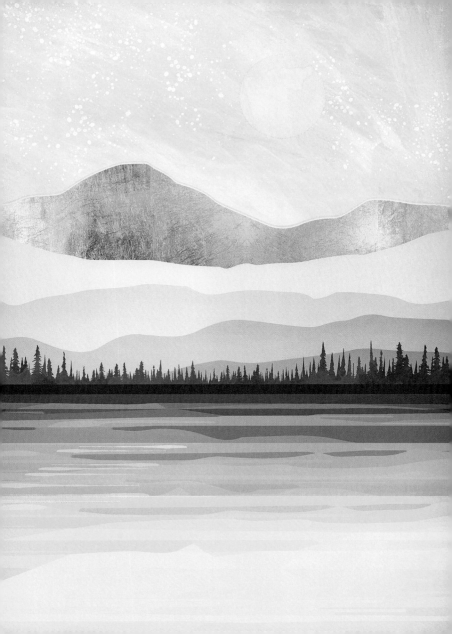

* **Essential oil:** To aid this meditation, mix one to two drops of Roman chamomile essential oil with a carrier oil and apply it to your forehead or behind your ears.

* **Ritual:** Sit quietly before starting this meditation and reflect on the times in your life when you have felt happy and fulfilled. Where were you? Who were you with? What were you doing?

✳ Become aware of the sounds that you can hear. Let your attention rest on the sounds close to you, within the same room.

Then let your attention wander beyond the room. What can you hear in the rest of the house? Let your attention rest on the sounds in the house for a while. What else can you hear?

Now let your attention wander beyond the house. What can you hear outside? Follow the sounds outside for a little while. Let your attention rest on the sounds outside your house. What else do you hear?

Then let your attention return to the room you are in, and let your focus rest on the sound of your own breath.

Inhaling, exhaling.

Settle deeper into your body with each breath, knowing that you are preparing to go on a journey, and that journey will be by boat.

You set out on a well-trodden path towards the lake, just as twilight creeps in and the sun makes way for the night. Even as the light fades, you feel safe and assured as you make the short walk. You know nothing will harm you here. You see the first playful stars piercing the night sky, as the moon illuminates your path, showing you the way. It feels good to be alive!

Up ahead, you see a person holding a lantern waiting for you on the banks of the lake. You know it is the ferryman, and that he is expecting you. Before you enter the boat, he waits. This is the moment you know you must choose your question, for later, out on the lake, you will be able to ask the ferryman this question. You pause – it is a big question about what gives your life meaning and you want some time to shape your question.

What is the question that is arising for you?

When your question is clear to you, you nod and the ferryman holds the boat steady. As you step in, you can hear the water lapping rhythmically against the wooden hull. You let your

attention rest on this and other sounds as they emerge. You become aware that the darkness enhances even soundless sounds, as a bird flies silently across the velvet skies.

With every oar stroke the ferryman takes you deeper into the darkness at the centre of the lake. In the silence of the night your breathing moves in time with each stroke of the oars. You can feel the coolness of your breath enter your nose as you inhale at the same moment the blades of the oars break the surface of the still lake. The ferry man drives the boat forward and you exhale fully into the dark night air in time with the oars as they leaves the water. Inhale again as the blades break the surface of the still lake, the boat moving forward as you exhale fully at the same time as the oars leave the water.

You count twenty strokes, inhaling and exhaling as the ferryman continues the journey. You feel safe and know you are exactly where you are supposed to be.

When the time comes, the ferryman stops rowing and rests the oars inside the boat. You know it is time to ask him your question, the question you brought with you as you climbed into the boat. You ask the ferryman your question and wait for his reply.

It makes perfect sense.

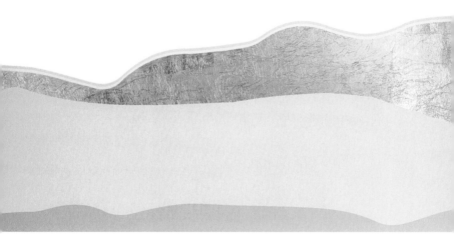

You enjoy the thoughtful silence as the boat silently slips back to shore. Back on the banks of the lake, you thank the ferryman for his guidance. He hands you a lantern so that you can retrace your steps back home.

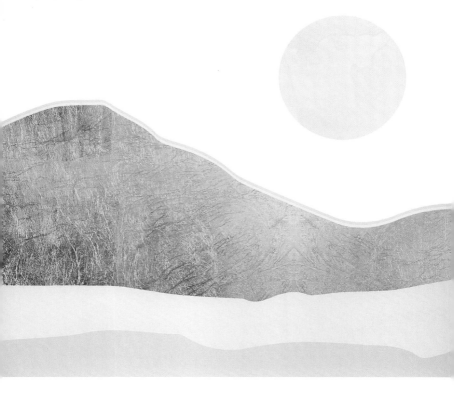

Coming home

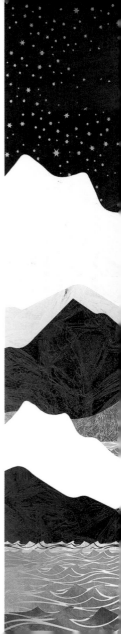

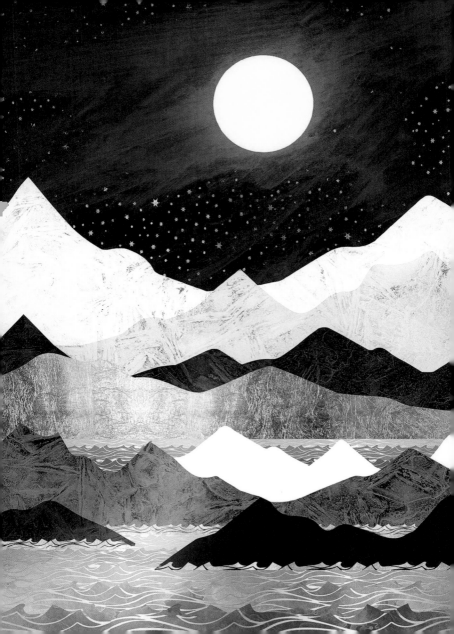

✳ Essential oil: Mix one to two drops of jasmine essential oil with a carrier oil and apply it to your sacral chakra (an energy centre located at the lower abdomen, below your navel).

✳ Ritual: Sit in a comfortable cross-legged position. Place your hands on your knees with your back straight and your chins slightly tucked in. Close your eyes, and take your attention inwards. Your attention can simply follow your breath inwards. Just let your attention rest instinctively at your centre, wherever this is for you.

Now, with your hands on your knees and your attention inwards, at your centre, begin to make a circle with your upper body. Circle your upper body in front of you; pass through the centre, as the energy of the circle naturally flows in front of you again. Circle four or five times in one direction and then four or five times in the other direction. If you enjoy this and want to do more, you can.

When you are ready to stop, return to your neutral position and place your left hand on your abdomen and your right hand on top of your left. Breathe deeply, feeling your belly rise beneath your hands with each inhale and fall with each exhale. Take five to eight breaths here, whatever feels comfortable to you. You can remain in this position now as you begin the meditation.

✳ As you begin this meditation, tell yourself that it is time to let go of other matters for the moment.

This is your time, your space, just for you.

There is nothing you need to do here; you don't need to try hard.

Sit in a comfortable cross-legged position, with your back straight and your chin slightly tucked in. Place your left hand on your abdomen and place your right hand on top of your left. Focus your attention on your breathing – in, and out.

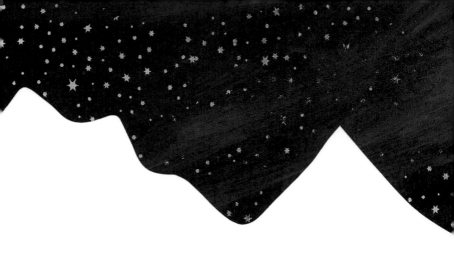

You are going on a journey. It is
a journey back to you, a journey
to remember your essence.

If you ever feel lost along the way, simply come back to your
breath – nothing else is required, no effort is needed here.

You begin your journey at the top of a beautiful staircase.
You admire the staircase, noticing what it is made from and
how solid it is. There are ten steps and, although they lead
into darkness, you know there is something precious for you
to discover there.

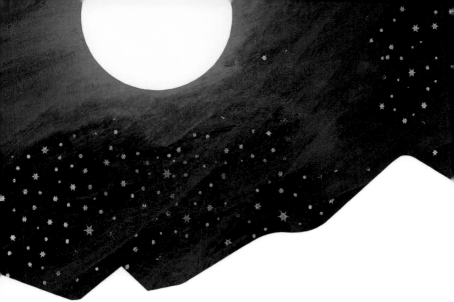

You take the first step and begin to count down slowly: ten, you breathe deeply and feel the weight of your body. Nine, you take another breath and another step. Eight, sinking down slowly as you breathe deeply. Seven, your mind feels calm as you take another step down. Six, with every step you feel calm and more relaxed. Five, you are even more deeply relaxed, taking another step down. Four, you sink even deeper now. Three, you relax even further with this step. Two, you're almost floating now. One, you step down, light as a feather, into an exquisite chamber infused with a peaceful and radiant light. As you arrive at this place of pure living beauty, every part of your body and being feels completely relaxed.

Coming home

You gaze in awe at the living beauty of your surroundings. Enveloped by the warm luminosity, you begin to realize that this is your own dwelling, a place at your core that is essentially you.

You walk towards a large ornate mirror in the centre of the chamber and stand before it. Without need, expectation or desire, you stand before the mirror and wait for an image or a message to appear. You trust the message, however it comes, and allow it to sink into your entire being.

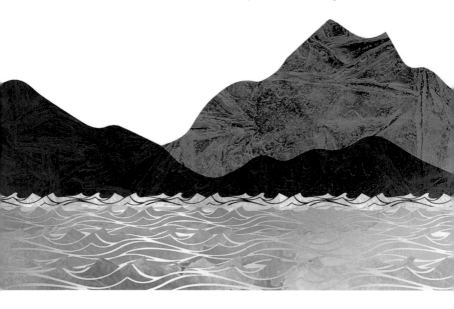

You are bathed in peace and tranquillity, and know that you can return to this place at any time.

This is home. Stay for as long as you like.

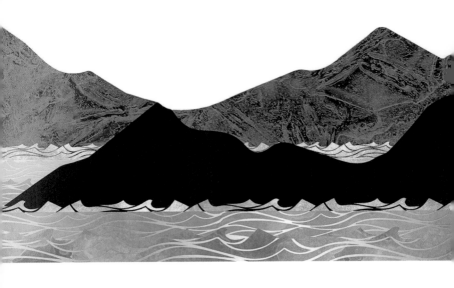

Coming home

You're OK, it's OK

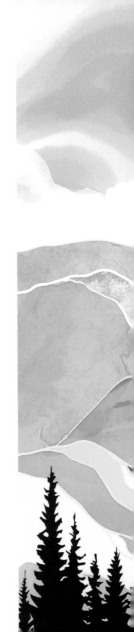

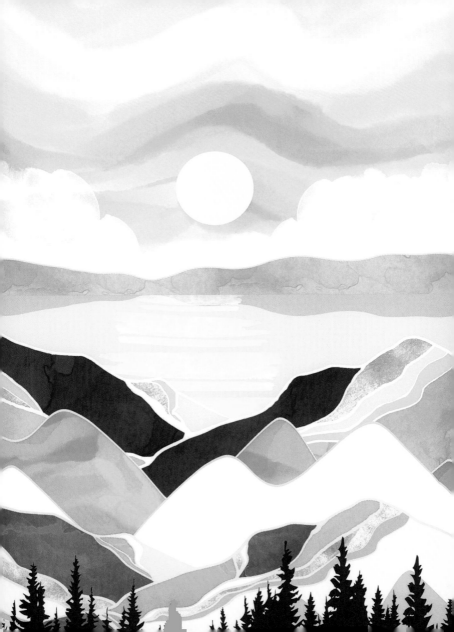

✳ Essential oil: Mix one to three drops of manuka essential oil with a carrier oil and apply it to the crown of your head.

✳ Ritual: This ritual is designed to be completed after the meditation. When you go to bed this evening, focus your intention on dreaming and on remembering your dreams. Put a notebook and pen by your bed; when you wake up in the morning, note down anything you remember from your dreams. What does it mean to you?

✳ Find a comfortable place to sit where you won't be disturbed. Turn the lights down and, once you are sitting in the most comfortable position for you, take a deep breath and sink into your body as you exhale.

Let yourself picture the night sky. See its deep darkness of the and bring it closer to you.

As you bring the night sky closer to you, you begin to see the stars. You draw the sky and the stars closer to you until you are the sky and the stars.

You let yourself travel in the expansiveness of space. You can see the celestial galaxies, created over a period of time of such magnitude that it is impossible for the human mind to truly comprehend their ancientness. You are in awe that you have a place here, that you are a part of it, this expansive universe, which goes beyond your imagination and yet exists.

You take a breath, knowing there is nothing to fear here.

You're OK and it's OK.

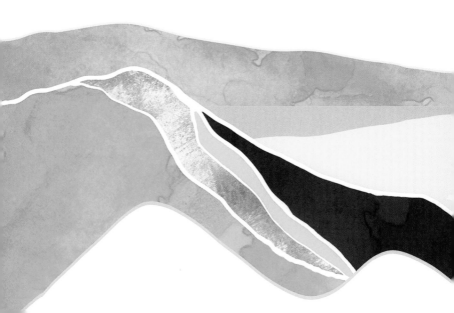

In this space, you understand that everything has its place and you are a part of it. As you float in the expansiveness of space, where time has no time at all, you think about your earthly struggles. You recall a struggle you have that has been particularly challenging. From this viewpoint, you consider your struggle with a loving, fresh perspective. How different your struggle seems from here!

You realize that you can let go of the struggle. It really is that simple after all.

You're OK and it's OK.

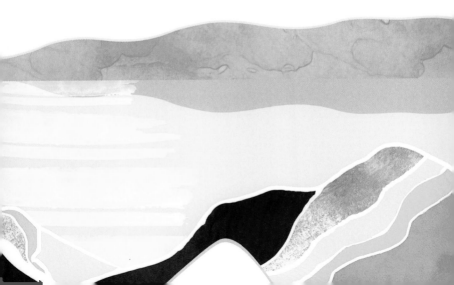

As you float in the expansiveness of space, you connect to a place that feels like home within you, a safe place that you can return to at any time, whenever you need to. Your home within you allows you to connect to yourself while being connected to the entire Universe. You realize you are within the Universe and the Universe is within you.

As you have this realization, the corners of your mouth turn upwards into a smile. Feel the smile radiate into your heart and down into your belly. Send the smile out beyond you, back into the Universe, as you return to the here and now, full of gratitude for the life of which you are a part.

Take a breath and place your right hand on your heart. Let the gratitude expand in your heart. Keeping your right hand on your heart, place your left hand on your belly and feel the gratitude radiate through your entire being.

There is so much to be grateful for. This breath in this moment. This day in this life. This body, just as it is. The people who love you and whom you love. This home, a warm and safe place to live. The abundance of food and plentiful water. The animals and nature that support you unconditionally.

Energy protection

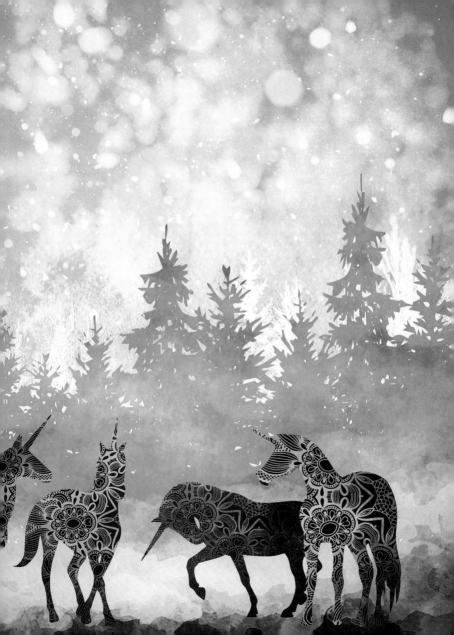

✳ **Essential oil:** Help promote a strong energetic backbone by diluting one to three drops of birch essential oil with a carrier oil and applying it along the spine or over the lower back.

✳ **Ritual:** Every day we are exposed to energy that is not our own. It comes from the people around us, advertising, weather, music, television, media, Wi-Fi and much more. We can't see this energy, but we are sensitive to it, and it can sometimes disturb the balance of our own energy without us even realizing this has happened. This is why you might feel better when you leave the city and go to the ocean, where the energy is more soothing to the system. Most people can't get to the ocean every day, so another option is to wear a protective crystal called Shungite, either as a pendant or a bracelet.

* This is a meditation to help clear any negative energy from the day. You can do this meditation lying down in a relaxed and comfortable position. Allow yourself to feel fully supported by the earth beneath you.

You are safe and grounded.

Let your breath settle.

Now, imagine a point of light about 2.5cm (1 inch) from your nose. Keeping it the same distance away from you, allow this light to travel over your chin and throat.

The light then travels across your chest from right to left, spending some time over your heart area and making sure this area is well protected.

Let the light travel down your left arm, over your hand, underneath your palm and then along the inside of your arm and up to your armpit.

The light then travels back across your chest and down your right arm, over your right hand and then moves under your palm, inside your arm and up to your armpit.

You then allow the light to spread across your entire torso. Over your hips and down the front of your thighs. Let the light travel over your calves, and then your feet.

Now let the light go beyond your feet and travel into the earth below.

Deep, deep, deeper down, right down into the core of the earth.

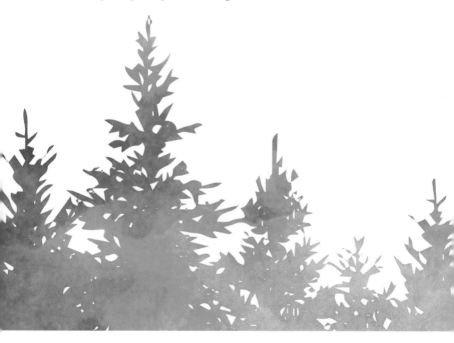

Then, drawing directly from her source, you bring the earth's energy up, up, up, allowing it to travel over the back of your heels, the backs of your calves, over your hips and lower back.

You let the energy travel up your spine, pausing at the back of your neck and ensuring this area is well protected.

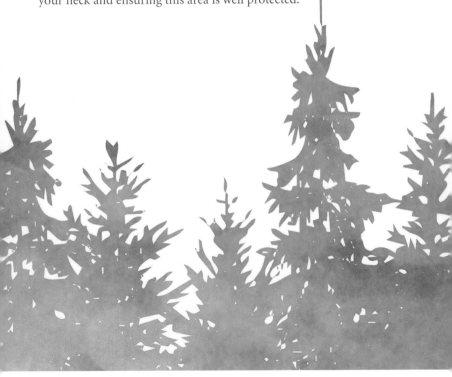

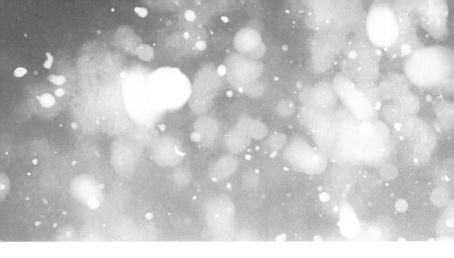

Allow the energy to travel over the back of your head and then, resting for a moment at the top of your head, send the energy from the earth up to the heights of the heavens.

A golden light showers down from the sky. Softly infusing every cell of your body with protective golden light.

Feel the light pouring like a golden liquid through your core and down through your feet.

This golden light goes back into the earth, drawing on her powerful core energy that is billions and billions of years old.

This majestic force covers your entire body and comes to rest at your third eye.

Here is where you know the truth that you are fully protected, and you have all the resources you need.

The energy seals at the top of your head. Imagine small psychic attacks coming towards you. Notice them bouncing off your energetic protection.

Now picture medium psychic attacks coming towards you. Notice them bouncing off, making no dent in your protection.

Then call on four black unicorns,
your final layer of protection.

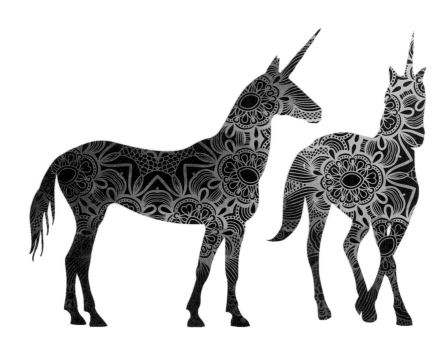

As they come into your awareness, you see that each unicorn is utterly jet black, with a coat that gleams like satin over its muscular flanks. The unicorns' dark eyes are fierce, and each of their horns is deadly sharp, but you know they are here for you, and their sole purpose is to protect you, not befriend you.

They are truly magnificent creatures, and they are your guardians.

Place one black unicorn facing outwards in front of you. Place a second black unicorn facing outwards to the right of you. Place your third black unicorn facing outwards to the left of you. Finally, place the last black unicorn facing outwards behind you.

As the unicorns surround you, you feel the immense power of their protection. You know that you are blessed and that the unicorns will be with you whenever you need them. You feel ready for the most peaceful sleep, and so you drift off.

Finding your way

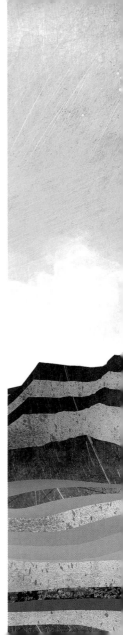

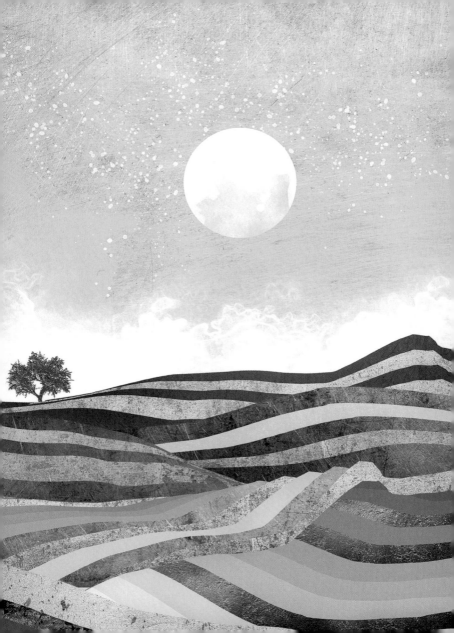

* **Essential oil:** To guide you during this meditation, add some ginger essential oil to a diffuser. Use just one to two drops, as this is a stimulating oil.

* **Ritual:** Before you begin, turn off your devices and arrange your space in such a way that you feel totally relaxed and comfortable. Wear some loose clothes and, if you need them, put on some socks to keep your feet warm. You might like to have a wrap or blanket nearby, too. Close the curtains, turn the lights down and light some candles if you wish.

  Sit in a relaxed position and, on a fresh page in your journal, write a list of the areas of your life you enjoy taking responsibility for. Let the list flow from the smallest area to the biggest, leaving no stone unturned. Next, write a list of any area that you avoid taking responsibility for. Be kind to yourself rather than critical, but also be honest about the areas you are avoiding. When you have finished, put your journal to one side. Nothing more is needed at this time; you are doing great.

✳ This is a meditation to help you find your way when you are feeling lost, directionless or lacking in purpose. There is nothing you need to do now except sit or lie quietly and comfortably, and simply relax.

Take a deep breath in through your nose, hold it for just a moment and then exhale deeply. Take another deep breath through your nose, hold it for just a moment and then exhale deeply. Once more, breathe in through your nose, hold it for just a moment and then exhale deeply.

During this visualization you will be protected by a guide. This might be a friend, a loved one, an animal, an angel or a spirit guide. Begin by inviting your guide to be alongside you now; know that they are always there for you, supporting and protecting you.

Imagine you are surrounded by a protective white light. With every inhale you will let more of this powerful light into your being.

Start at your feet and imagine that you are inhaling the light into your feet. Exhale. Now, inhale the light into your knees. Exhale. Inhale the light into your hips. Exhale. Inhale the light into your stomach. Exhale. Inhale the light into your chest.

Exhale. Inhale the light into your heart. Exhale. Inhale the light into your throat. Exhale. Inhale the light into your mind. Exhale. Inhale the light into the crown of your head. Exhale. Inhale the light into the back of your neck. Exhale. Inhale the light into your spine. Exhale. Inhale the light into your lower back. Exhale. Inhale the light into the palms of your hands. Exhale. Inhale the light into your legs. Exhale. Inhale the light into the soles of your feet. Exhale.

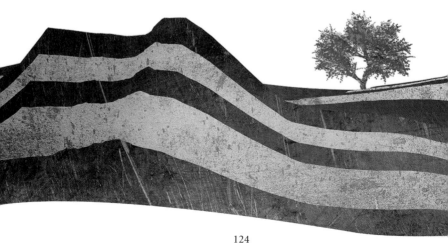

Continue to inhale the white, protective light into the soles of your feet and the palms of your hands, letting the light shimmer and pulsate. Send the light to any parts of you that need it. Experience the gently undulating wave of protective white light as it travels through your body. Rest here for a moment. When you are ready, bring your palms together, with your thumbs touching the space between your eyebrows, and give thanks to your guide for always being alongside you.

Now that you are completely relaxed, you are going to go on a journey.

Your journey begins on a path at the edge of a beautiful bamboo forest nestled at the foot of some ancient mountains.

The breeze ripples through the swaying stalks of bamboo and the sound invites you to enter. Through the tall, thick, tightly packed bamboo, the path is clear and easy to follow, and so you step into the forest.

Shafts of sunlight fall through the canopy, dancing between the leaves and welcoming you into the forest.

As you move deeper into the forest, where there is no breeze, the silence is total. You stand for a moment, enveloped in the silence. You can feel the life force of the forest pulsating as it transmits its medicinal, life-giving energy into you. In this moment you know that you are at one with the forest and you feel a profound sense of peace.

As you walk on, you begin to hear the sound of flowing water. You can tell the water is guiding you, and you walk in the direction of the sound. As you walk, you can feel a carpet of bamboo leaves under your feet, and you enjoy the connection to the earth as you let the gentle sound of the water call you on.

Emerging through the dark green bamboo, you begin to see flashes of turquoise as a small stream of clear mountain water makes itself known to you. You follow the stream until you reach a clearing where the water cascades down a short rocky slope into a beautiful emerald-green lotus pool. You watch the minute crystals of water dance like jewels in the air as the water flows into the lotus pool. The water comes to rest serenely before leaving the pool on the other side and continuing its journey.

The pool is inviting, and there are some rocks by the water where you can sit. The rocks are warm from the sun and covered with a rich green velvety moss. You walk to the largest of the rocks and take a seat on it. It is as if the rock were made just for you to sit on. The moss forms a cushion and the rock cradles your body and holds you steady. From this place you can clearly see a constellation of pink and white lotus flowers in the water. Their vivid blooms rise proudly from the muddy depths, knowing this is their place.

You sit here for a few minutes in silence, listening to the sounds of the water, watching red and blue dragonflies flit between the lotus flowers, your heart full of joy.

You become aware of another presence and see a beautiful blue heron standing on the opposite side of the pool. Its eyes are fixed on yours, and you are enthralled by the beauty and presence of this magnificent bird. You sense that the blue heron has come to communicate with you; it is a messenger. You are being given guidance on the direction of your life.

Whatever you need to know will be provided. You appreciate the importance of this moment and open your heart, ready to receive the wisdom that is intended for you.

In the space between you and the heron the message is conveyed and you receive it wholeheartedly. You feel honoured to have been visited by such an important messenger and express your gratitude wordlessly through your eyes to the blue heron. The bird shifts its weight on the stone, expands its wings and, as silently as it arrived, takes flight through the forest.

You sit for a moment longer, simply integrating into your being the message that was brought for you.

When you are ready, you rise from your mossy spot on the rock, move gently back onto the path and walk purposefully, knowing that you have the power to direct your own destiny, as you make your way back to the edge of the forest where you first stepped onto the path.

Closing ritual: When you have completed the meditation, take a moment to write your message in your journal. Then go back to the original lists you made and explore any connections between the message you received and the lists you made. Write down any observations and insights before you go to bed, and then let your dreams guide you further as you sleep.

Meeting your guides

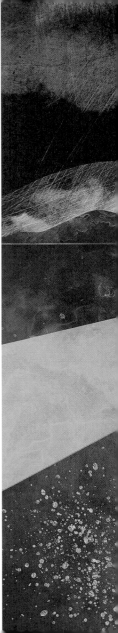

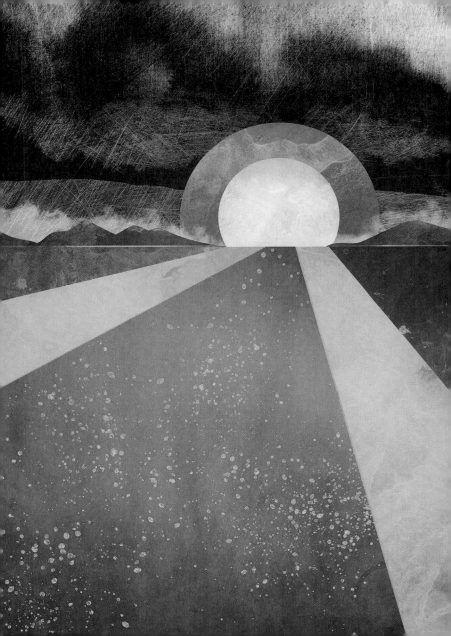

✳ Essential oil: Add ten to twelve drops of juniper berry essential oil to a small spray bottle of water (60ml/2fl oz). Shake well and mist your room both before the meditation and before you go to bed.

✳ Ritual: Create a simple altar. An altar is personal and can be as effortless as a stone you collected from a beach or a collection of items with significance to you, such as a photograph, a candle and some crystals. You can bring the outdoors in for your altar, adding a seasonal leaf or bloom.

How you use the altar is up to you. You might touch the stone as you leave the house and say an affirmation, or sit by your altar for a couple of minutes in the morning and set an intention for the day ahead.

✳ Sit in front of your altar or hold an item in your right hand
that you connect with and that has a meaning or special
significance to you.

Place your right hand in your left hand and let your arms and
shoulders relax. Lower your gaze or close your eyes, then turn
your attention to your heart space. If it helps, take a breath now
and connect with your heart.

If your mind is busy, let it be; the mind is designed to think.
If you find yourself getting distracted at any time by your
thoughts, simply come back to your breathing and notice the
steady rhythm of your inhale and exhale, which is always
available to you.

On the next inhale, let your attention travel with your breath
from your heart chakra up to your third eye chakra – the space
between your eyes. Take three deliberate breaths: in through
your right nostril, up into your third eye and out through your
left nostril. You may wonder if your breath can move in this
way, simply direct your breath and watch it travel in through
your right nostril and out through your left.

On the next inhale, let your attention travel from your third eye to your crown chakra – the point at the very top of your head. Take three deliberate breaths: in through your nose and up to your crown chakra.

Continue now with your regular breath, keeping your attention on your crown chakra.

From your crown chakra, imagine a beam of golden light that connects you with the heavens.

This beam of light begins to expand, getting wider and wider until, very simply, you can travel through it, finding yourself enveloped by the gorgeous golden glow.

You travel through the beam of golden light until it is time to step off. You step safely through the beam of light into another dimension, knowing that the beam of light will guide you back when it is time.

Standing in front of you is a group of wise elders. Some you recognize, others are unfamiliar to you. There are sages and shamans, angels and warriors, animals and long-lost friends. Each stands there for you, meeting you with love and understanding in their eyes. They understand the triumphs and tribulations, the heartbreaks and successes. They understand what you have had to overcome to be here, in this moment right now, because they have always been with you.

You approach them one by one, connecting eye to eye and heart to heart, before kneeling in front of them. You bow your head and hold out your hands, and each guide gives you a blessing. It may be in the form of words, an object or by touching your head, or it might be another type of message. You receive each blessing with an open heart.

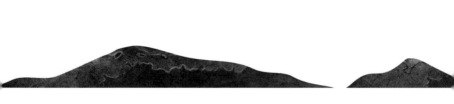

The final guide you meet invites you to stand. They state that as you have received these blessings, you can leave anything you came with that no longer serves you with your guides. Should you require it in the future, you may return and collect it. You consider for a moment what it is that no longer serves you and feel it leaving your body.

It is time to leave your guides, but you know you leave filled with blessings and an appreciation that they are always with you.

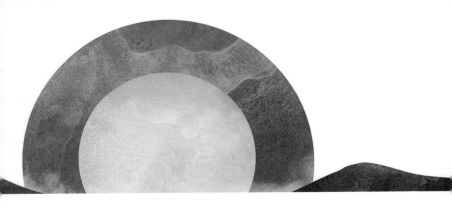

You turn towards the bright golden light, step back into it and feel yourself enveloped by the gorgeous golden glow.

You travel back down into your physical body as the golden glow narrows to a beam of light. You begin to draw the beam of light in through your crown chakra, down through your third eye and seal it within your heart.

You rest, feeling rooted and absorbing the blessings you have received. You give silent thanks to your guides who support you and watch over you.

Meeting your guides

Ocean waves

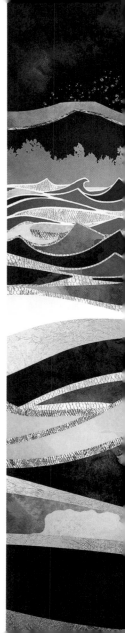

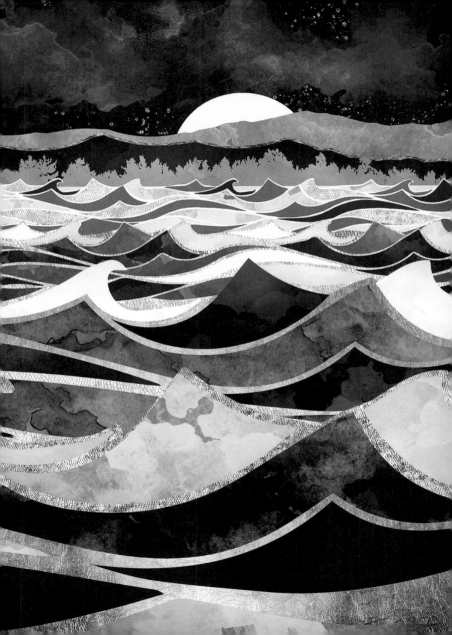

✳ Essential oil: For emotional connection, add some ylang-ylang essential oil to a diffuser or mix one to three drops with a carrier oil and apply it over your heart.

✳ Ritual: After your meditation, you could take a warm bath. For an even more restorative soak, mix one to two drops of ylang-ylang essential oil in one cup of Epsom salts or coarse sea salt, then dissolve the mix in your bathwater (alternatively, you can use the salts with no essential oil). Light a candle or some incense, lie back and relax.

✳ Find a place to sit where you won't be disturbed. You are going to be relaxed but remain awake during this meditation. Turn the lights down and sit comfortably, making any final adjustments in order to feel completely comfortable. Take a deep breath in through your nose, and as you exhale, make a sound – whatever wants to come out. With every exhale, let everything go.

Inhale and make a sound on the exhale, letting everything go. One more inhale and let the sound come out with the exhale, relaxing and letting your entire body sink into the floor. Feel your body being totally supported and let go a little more.

Bring to mind your favourite beach, and begin to hear the sound of the waves as they come to shore. Let your breath be in harmony with the waves as they flow in and out, in and out. Smell the salt in the air as your breath continues to harmonize with the waves as they flow in and out, in and out.

As you breathe in harmony with the ocean waves, let go of trying too hard to do this. Let it happen naturally, just as it does in nature and within you.

Begin now to scan your body from your head to your feet. Starting with your head, eyes, jaw and neck, becoming aware of any emotions you might be feeling.

Move down towards your shoulders, chest and heart, noticing any feelings that are present.

Continue to scan your arms, hands and abdomen, feeling what you feel as you scan down your thighs, calves and feet.

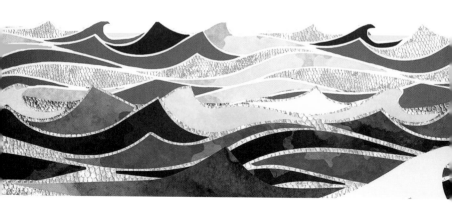

All the time your breathing is like a wave, naturally flowing in and flowing out.

Now return to an area of your body that would benefit from your care and attention, an area where you felt some emotion during the body scan. Don't think too hard about this, but let your instincts guide you. You will know just where to rest your attention. As you let your attention rest on this part of your body, begin to feel the sensation that is here. What do you notice? Is there a temperature, hot or cold? Is there a sensation of emptiness or fullness? Is it heavy or light, sharp or smooth? Or something entirely different?

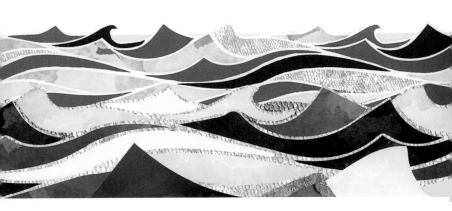

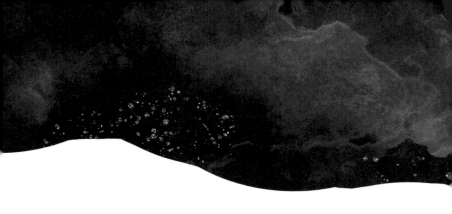

Play with the quality of the sensation. Can you stretch it? Can you intensify it? Can you soften it? Can you bring light to it? Can you begin to dissolve it? Stay curious to your experience and play with it until you are ready to simply give it all back to the ocean. Let it go and begin to breathe in harmony with the waves, flowing in and flowing out.

As you connect with your breath, feel the breeze dance on your skin, the sunlight warm on your face, and know all is well.

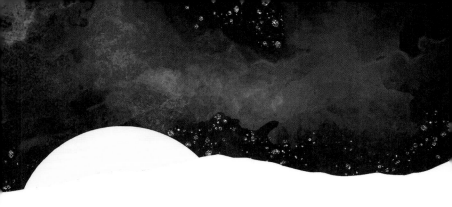

Lie or sit peacefully for as long as you wish, feeling your breathing in harmony with the ocean waves.

When you are ready, stretch your arms above your head and wriggle your jaw, letting go of any sound or yawns that want to come out.

Put your hands together at your heart centre and, in your own time, you can take yourself off for a peaceful night's sleep.

The inner journey

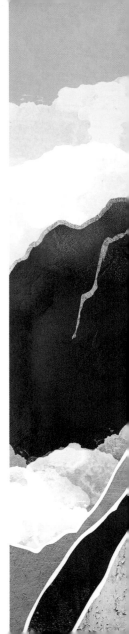

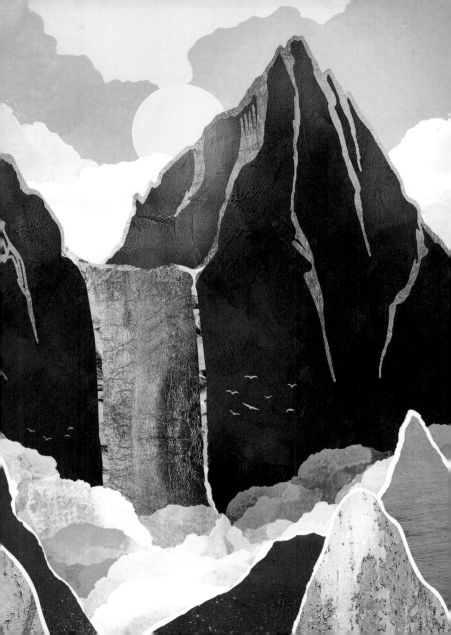

✳ Essential oil: For additional cleansing, inhale some lemongrass essential oil.

✳ Ritual: Switch off your devices, close the curtains and turn down the lights. Get settled in a comfortable place with your journal and a pen. Before you begin the meditation, write down anything that is on your mind which may distract you or get in the way of your meditation this evening. Then put your journal and any distractions aside, knowing that you can attend to these things tomorrow.

✳ This is your time. A time for total relaxation and inner stillness. Take a moment to make sure you are warm enough, and that you are seated in a comfortable position. Support your knees with cushions if needed.

Begin by placing your left hand on your left knee with your palm facing upwards. Connect your thumb and middle finger and let your hand lightly rest in this position. Now place your index and middle finger of your right hand in the space between your eyebrows. Massage this area, known as the third eye, in an anticlockwise direction and then in a clockwise direction. Keeping your two fingers in the space between your brows, let your thumb rest over your right nostril and your ring finger rest over your left nostril. Your little finger can simply relax. You are going to practise some yogic breathing. If at any time you need more air, simply sip it in through your mouth.

Close your right nostril with your thumb. Inhale through your left nostril for a count of four. Close your left nostril, pause, open your right nostril and exhale for a count of four. Pause. Inhale through your right nostril. Close your right nostril, pause and then open your left nostril and exhale for a count of four. Pause. That was one cycle. Repeat the cycle four more times ending with the final exhale on your left nostril.

Now place your right hand on your right knee, with your palm facing upwards. Connect your thumb and middle finger and breath normally for a moment, noticing the effect of your practice so far.

Imagine a small flickering flame at the base of your spine. Inhale at the base of your spine using your breath to encourage the flame to grow. Let the flame rise up through your spinal column, vertebra by vertebra; feel your backbone strengthen as the fire rises. Take your time, controlling the intensity and pace of the flame with your breath. Inhale as the flame enters your neck and travels over the back of your head. Exhale and let the flame dance at the top of your head. Inhale and watch as it transforms into molten golden light. Exhale and let the golden light pour over your forehead and run through your throat. Inhale and follow the golden light as it fills your chest, and exhale as it flows into your heart. Inhale as the golden light liquifies in your stomach, a pure, bright, golden light. Exhale, letting the shimmering, molten light gather at the base of your spine. Inhale as you watch the golden light returning to the place of your flame, the fire and light merging as one, fuelling your inner spirit and strengthening your resolve. Exhale and bring your hands to pray, your thumbs touching your heart. Say your name to yourself and give thanks to you for all that you are.

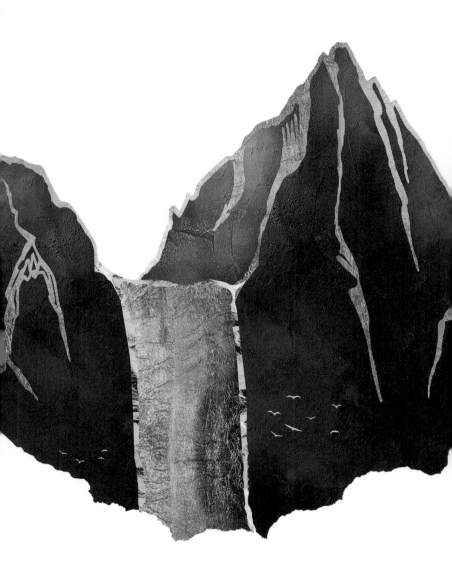

151

The inner journey

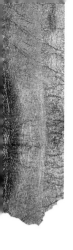

Now it is time to leave the external world behind and go on an inner journey. A journey to a place of deep inner stillness.

You notice that you are standing on a beautiful sandy beach just as the sun is preparing to set slowly over the horizon. You feel a warm, gentle, salty breeze on your skin and see the soft pink light of the setting sun. The sand feels warm under your feet; you can sink into the softness as you listen to the gentle rolling rhythm of the waves lapping against the shore.

You feel relaxed and at ease with yourself and the world. You have this beautiful beach all to yourself, and all the time in the world.

You become aware that you have a small rucksack on your back.

You listen to the relaxing sound of the ocean, the rhythm of the waves, steady and reassuring as they roll in and out; there is no rush or hurry here. You feel drawn to the ocean and begin to walk slowly towards the water's edge.

There is a small rowing boat waiting for you, tied to the shore with a strong rope. You pause for a moment, glancing up as a bird glides effortlessly above you. Walking into the warm, clear blue water, you step into the boat, bringing your rucksack with you.

When you are ready, untie the rope and let it go.

The natural currents of the ocean guide you gently away from the beach. Your boat drifts and rocks ever so gently in the water.

The ocean water around you sparkles with a soft rose-pink in the glow of the low, setting sun. In front of you, a small island comes into view.

Your boat brings you closer to the island, effortlessly moving through the water until it comes gently to rest on the shore.

You have arrived.

Remembering your rucksack, you step out of the boat onto warm white sand. You look around and take in your surroundings, in awe of the beauty of nature around you. Within a few steps of the shoreline there are brilliantly coloured flowers and exotic birds dancing in the trees, chatting away to each other.

This place has a very special energy that makes you feel relaxed, but also curious to explore. You are completely present and soaking up the gentle, luminous energy of this beautiful place.

You feel at peace.

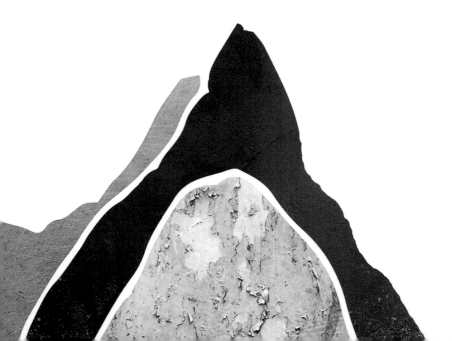

You notice an opening between the palm trees. In the centre of this opening there is a narrow path that leads towards a small hill.

You follow the path as it meanders between the trees until it begins to follow the gentle incline of the hill. Step by step, moment by moment, you feel safer and happier as you walk the path knowing all is well. As you get closer to the top of the hill, a small ancient building comes into view. You reach the summit and are met by two large wooden doors: the gatekeepers of this sacred place. You place your hands on the doors, feeling the rough wooden texture under your palms, and push the heavy doors which open with ease.

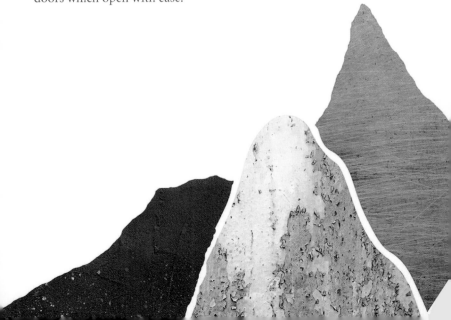

Inside is a space that feels familiar to you, like the memory of a pleasant dream or a place you visited as a child.

You see a magnificent stained-glass window at the end of the room. Evening sunlight pours into the space through this kaleidoscope of colour, illuminating the room like a cathedral. You are guided into the room by a force that you trust, and this makes you feel safe and at peace.

You stand at the very heart of the room, with prisms of colour dancing around you. Before you there is a table, and you now know why you have come. You place your rucksack on the table. The rucksack contains a heavy load, one that you no longer need to bear. You take out the contents of the rucksack and reverently leave it on the table. There was a reason why you carried this load at the time, and you feel thankful for all the lessons you have learned by doing so. You express your gratitude for having been guided here, to this moment right now, where you can let go and leave this heavy load behind. As you let go, leaving your heavy load in this sacred space, your mind seems to expand. You feel timeless...vast...empty...relaxed.

You enjoy this experience of inner silence. When thoughts arise, you simply let them go and return your awareness to the prisms of light dancing around you.

Now it is time to make your way back home. You pick up your empty backpack, and feel light, clear and happy.

You turn to leave the room, pushing open the doors back to the path, and are welcomed by a sky shimmering red, gold, pink and orange as the sun follows your descent back down the path to the palm trees, back to your boat, knowing in your heart that you can return any time you wish.

You arrive back at the palm trees and the sandy beach. Your boat is waiting for you, just where you left it.

Walk to the water's edge and climb into the boat.

You feel relaxed and secure. You know that your boat will bring you home safely.

Your journey is effortless and calm. You feel light and clear as you relax and allow the current to guide you.

You arrive at the beach, step out of the boat and onto the sand. You are home.

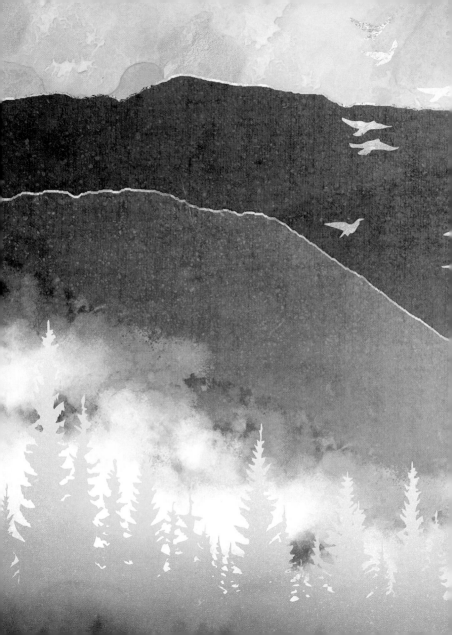

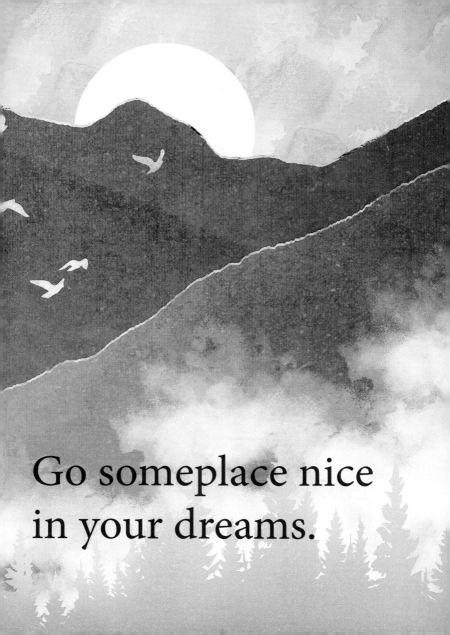

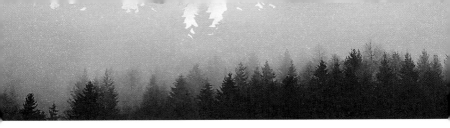

About the author

Danielle North has a history as a successful executive coach in the corporate industry, working with top-level executives at companies such as HSBC, McKinsey, Unilever and SAP. She has more than 15 years' experience working with leaders in 20 different countries. After learning that goals and ambitions could be just as happily and successfully achieved when simply allowing the body and mind to pause, she adapted her coaching style with both personal and corporate clients to flow rather than fight against the ups and downs of life.

www.pauseglobal.com

www.facebook.com/pauseglobal

@pauseglobal_

@pauseglobal_